ADVANCES IN RESEARCH ON DOWN SYNDROME

Edited by **Subrata Dey**

Advances in Research on Down Syndrome
http://dx.doi.org/10.5772/intechopen.68260
Edited by Subrata Dey

Contributors

Eugene Yu, Zhuo Xing, Yichen Li, Garrett Kaas, Annie Pao, Fatih Hilmi Çetin, Sevde Afife Ersoy, Hasan Ali Güler, Anna Conti, Antonella Izzo, Nunzia Mollo, Lucio Nitsch, Rita Cicatiello, Rita Genesio, Simona Paladino, Felipe Garcia-Vallejo, Alejandra Rodriguez, Meliza Santiago Ospina, Julio Cesar Montoya, Camila Azcarate, Adalberto Sanchez, Jose Maria Satizabal, Dominic Iliescu, Dragusin Roxana, Honey Heussler, Jasneek Chawla, Colin J. McMahon, Louise Morrison, Sophie Duignan

Published by InTech
Janeza Trdine 9, 51000 Rijeka, Croatia

Publishing Process Manager Iva Simcic
Technical Editor SPi Global
Cover InTech Design team

First published January, 2018
Printed in Croatia
Legal deposit, Croatia: National and University Library in Zagreb

Additional hard copies can be obtained from orders@intechopen.com

Advances in Research on Down Syndrome, Edited by Subrata Dey
p. cm.
Print ISBN 978-953-51-3762-7
Online ISBN 978-953-51-3763-4

Meet the editor

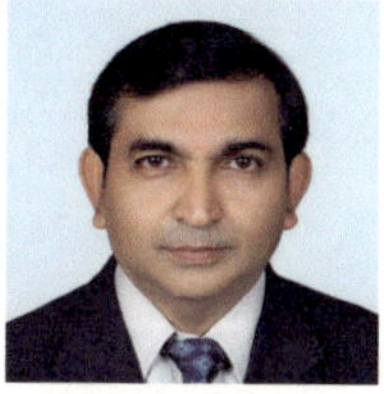

Subrata Dey is a professor of Biotechnology and pro-vice chancellor at Maulana Abul Kalam Azad University of Technology (formerly West Bengal University of Technology). His major research interests are molecular genetics of Down syndrome, identification of genes involved in the development of congenital heart disease and Alzheimer's disease in both Down syndrome and healthy individuals. His group also studies the mechanism of radiation-induced genomic instability and radioprotection, genetics of dental diseases and antioxidants. Prof. Dey has been teaching courses in Genetics, Molecular Biology and Developmental Biology and is the author of many scientific papers .He has also edited four books on Down syndrome. Prof. Dey is the founding director of Centre for Genetic Studies and has developed a free online learning portal on Genetics and Biotechnology (www.genomegyan.com).

Contents

Preface

Down syndrome (DS) or trisomy 21 is the most frequent live born chromosomal aneuploidy in humans, characterized by an extra chromosome 21. Researchers have contributed significantly towards understanding the management and control of mental and physical disabilities associated with Down syndrome. Since mid-nineteenth century, Down syndrome research has progressed alongside and in response to more general scientific advances. These researches attempt to cover the aetiology, psychopathology, different types of diseases, treatment, prenatal screening and diagnosis, epidemiology, management and prevention of Down syndrome. Both *in vitro* and *in vivo* experiments are carried out to understand the molecular mechanism of origin of this aneuploidy. Many exciting areas are currently being investigated in relation to Down syndrome. A number of genes have been identified, which are putative candidates for phenotypic abnormalities in Down syndrome. The use of Down syndrome mouse model, which is segmental trisomy of homologous segment of human chromosome 21, has facilitated greatly the process of reverse genetic approach to explore the gene-protein relationship in Down syndrome individuals.

Thrust is being made in areas of research on functional neurogenomics and psychopathology for the management of cognitive and mental disabilities and behavioural disorders in individuals with Down syndrome. Studies performed both in humans and in animal models have shown that trisomy 21 leads to an imbalance of key cellular events, such as neuronal cell proliferation and differentiation. A reduced neuron number is found in the cortex, hippocampus and cerebellum of DS brain and are accompanied by impaired neuronal function leading to intellectual disability.

This book is organized into four sections. All sections include chapters on recent advances in research on Down syndrome. The editor endeavoured to keep the big picture and overarching philosophy of the review articles in focus while editing the text and illustrations for consistent use of scientific terminology.

The first section deals with chromosome engineering. The emergence of CRISPR/Cas9 facilitated chromosome editing techniques that may open up a new avenue to study human diseases associated with chromosomal abnormalities such as Down syndrome. With the addition of this technique, it is reasonable to predict that many important insights into Down syndrome will be revealed in the near future. Moreover, new knowledge on this disorder will be instrumental for developing therapeutic strategies for the treatment of Down syndrome individuals.

The second section discusses mental retardation and cognitive disabilities. The first chapter focuses on psychopathology in Down syndrome. Studies suggest that children with Down syndrome are at increased risk of psychopathologies, which include anxiety disorder, bipolar disorder, obsessive-compulsive disorder, autism, depression, conduct disorder and attention deficit hyperactivity disorder. Therefore, it is important to perform psychological evaluations of patients with Down syndrome during routine follow-ups. The second chapter focuses on functional neurogenomics, which is the interface between neuroscience knowledge and omics science data. Understanding the functional neurogenomics of Down syndrome brain emerges as a new scenario to partially overcome the cognitive disability through new prospective genomic therapies. The third chapter highlights the sleep disorders in Down syndrome, which are common and often overlooked problem in Down syndrome, particularly during childhood. This disorder affects the central nervous system, cardiovascular and metabolic systems, which ultimately lead to reduced quality of life.

The third section covers prenatal diagnosis, which reviews multiple screening methods for trisomy 21 foetuses. Down syndrome can be suspected during pregnancy by using genetic ultrasound method, which measures the nuchal translucency (NT) and is considered as the most important marker for the first trimester detection of Down syndrome foetus.

The concluding section focuses on diseases associated with Down syndrome. The association between Down syndrome and congenital heart disease, particularly atrioventricular septal defect (AVSD) that comprises 30 to 40% of all cardiac defects in Down syndrome. A routine cardiac screening of all new born babies with Down syndrome is recommended. Recent studies highlight a link between mitochondrial dysfunction and complex Down syndrome phenotype. It has been suggested that counteracting the mitochondrial defect in Down syndrome may improve the neurological phenotype and prevent Down syndrome–associated pathologies such as Alzheimer's disease, type 2 diabetes and obesity, thus providing a better quality of life for Down syndrome individuals and their families.

This book provides a concise yet comprehensive source of current information on Down syndrome. Research workers, scientists, medical graduates and paediatricians will find the book on Down syndrome as an excellent source for reference and review.

The editor wants to acknowledge the superb assistance of staff members and management of InTechOpen Publisher, in particular Ms. Iva Simcic, Publishing Process Manager, for coordination and editorial assistance. We are grateful to all contributing authors and scientists who made this book possible by providing valuable research and review articles. Finally, I would like to dedicate this book to children with Down syndrome who need our love and care to lead a healthy life.

Dr. Subrata Dey
Professor of Biotechnology,
Ex-Director, School of Biotechnology and Biological Sciences,
Pro-Vice chancellor, Maulana Abul Kalam Azad University of Technology,
Kolkata, West Bengal, India

Section 1

Chromosome Engineering in Down syndrome

Chapter 1

CRISPR/Cas9-Facilitated Chromosome Engineering to Model Human Chromosomal Alterations

Zhuo Xing, Yichen Li, Annie Pao, Garrett Kaas and
Y. Eugene Yu

Additional information is available at the end of the chapter

http://dx.doi.org/10.5772/intechopen.70897

Abstract

Rodents, particularly the mouse, have been used extensively for genetic modeling and analysis of human chromosomal alterations based on the syntenic conservations between the human and rodent genomes. In this article, we will discuss the emergence of CRISPR/Cas9-facilitated chromosome engineering techniques, which may open up a new avenue to study human diseases associated with chromosomal abnormalities, such as Down syndrome and cancer.

Keywords: human chromosomal anomalies, down syndrome, rodent models, chromosome engineering, CRISPR/Cas9

1. Introduction

Chromosomal alterations are a major cause of human disease. The presence of an extra copy of human chromosome 21 (Hsa21) leads to Down syndrome (DS). Due to the evolutionary conservation, orthologous regions of Hsa21 have been found in a limited number of discrete chromosomal segments in the genomes of other mammals, including mice and rats (**Figure 1**). These shared syntenies provide a treasure trove for genetic modeling as well as the mechanistic dissection of DS. The first rodent model generated for DS was a mutant mouse that carried an extra copy of mouse chromosome 16 (Mmu16), where many Hsa21 gene orthologs are located in this genomic region. However, given that the mouse was embryonic lethal, many groups soon turned their attention to the postnatally viable Ts65Dn mouse line, which carries an unbalanced derivative of an irradiation-induced translocation, Ts(17^{16})65Dn [1]. This extra chromosome contains the entire genomic region distal to *Mir155* on Mmu16 and a subcentromeric region on Mmu17, which is not

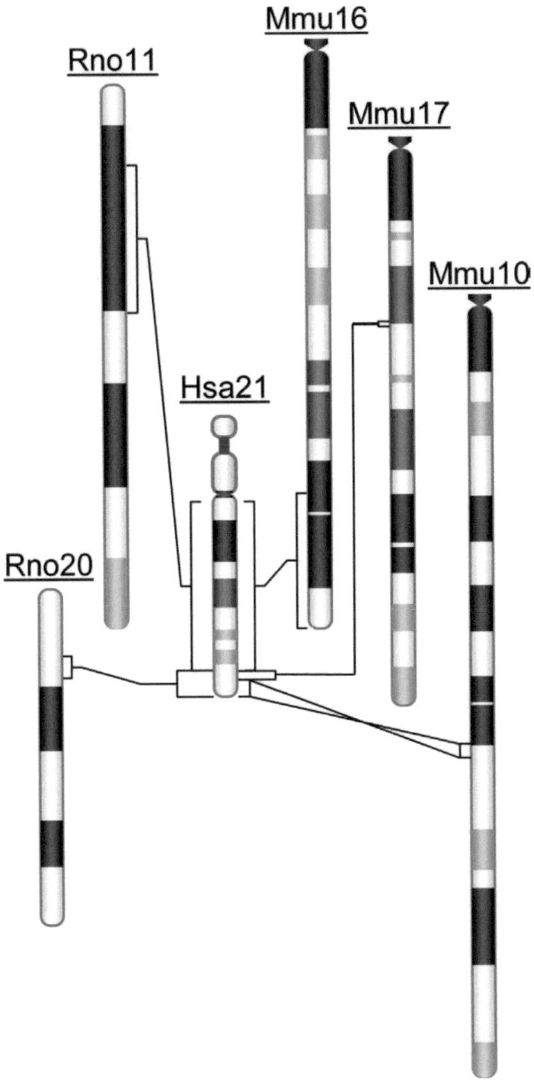

Figure 1. Schematic representation of Hsa21 and the syntenic regions on Mmu10, Mmu16, Mmu17, rat chromosome 11 (Rno11), and Rno20.

syntenic to Hsa21. Another attractive mouse model used by DS researchers is the transchromosomal strain, Tc1 [2], which carries a Hsa21. However, because Hsa21 was irradiated while being transferred to mouse ES cells through cell fusion, the Hsa21 in Tc1 mice carries several undesired genetic rearrangements, including deletions, duplications, and other rearrangements. Both Ts65Dn and Tc1 mice have been extensively characterized and show several phenotypic features similar to human DS despite the presence of secondary molecular aberrations [3]. In the recent years, the numbers of mouse mutants carrying rearranged Hsa21 syntenic regions has increased significantly due to the development of Cre/*loxP*-mediated chromosome engineering techniques. The most genetically accurate model among them is the line carrying triplications spanning the entirety of all Hsa21 syntenic regions, *Dp(10)1Yey/+;Dp(16)1Yey/+;Dp(17)1Yey/+* [4]. Phenotypic characterizations of this mutant revealed several important DS-related phenotypes, including heart defects and impaired cognitive function. Other engineered mouse mutants, which carry a triplication or deficiency of smaller Hsa21 syntenic regions [5, 6], have facilitated systematic genetic dissections of DS phenotypes. With the emergence of CRISPR/Cas9-facilitated genome editing, attempts have been made to further improve the efficiency of mammalian chromosome manipulations, whether it be deletions, duplications, inversions, or translocations [7–10], including those in Hsa21 syntenic regions.

2. The potential advantages of CRISPR/Cas9-facilitated chromosome engineering

Chromosome engineering enables the generations of deletions, duplications, inversions, and translocations in a particular genome of interest, which in turn are used as research tools for the genetic modeling and dissection of human diseases and disorders caused by chromosomal alterations. These models act as invaluable resources for researchers, aiding in the identification of causative genes and cellular mechanisms that underlie the presentation of clinical phenotypes associated with these genomic abnormalities, such as in DS. Using traditional Cre/*loxP*-mediated ES cell-based chromosome engineering approaches to generate chromosomal alterations requires a multistep process [11]. Such ES cells are limited to a few strains of mice, such as 129S5, and are not available for other rodent species, including rats. The most popular ES cell-based chromosome engineering procedure requires the use of ES cells carrying a null allele of *Hprt*.

For the aforementioned reasons, CRISPR/Cas9 may have the potential to play an important role in mammalian chromosome engineering, which complements the current approach. Specifically, it may offer opportunities to obtain mutants for other less commonly used animal models by direct zygote injection of the CRISPR/Cas9 components without involving ES cells [12–14]. This new approach may also facilitate chromosome engineering in mice from different strain backgrounds than those currently available with the Cre/*loxP*-mediated ES cell methods [7, 8]. Furthermore, it may lead to the generation of desired animal models more quickly. **Table 1** summarized the efficiencies of three types of structural variations, deletion, inversion, and duplication, in mouse [7, 8].

Although in Cre/*loxP*-mediated ES cell-based chromosome engineering, the size of the rearranged genomic regions is inversely correlated to the efficiency of generation of the desired chromosomal rearrangements, the same cannot be said for CRISPR/Cas9-facilitated chromosome engineering. Current data have not provided sufficient evidence to draw such a conclusion [7–9]. On the other hand, current data do suggest that chromosomal location and/or the endpoints of the fragment manipulated through CRISPR/Cas9 can influence the efficiency of genome engineering. In **Table 1**, the size of both the *Nox4-Grm5* and *Runx1-Cbr1* region is around 1.1 Mb; however, the efficiencies of generating F0 deletion mouse were 30 and 3%, respectively. Kraft et al. [9] also discovered the efficiency is variable among different loci. In addition, Boroviak et al. [8] concluded that the efficiencies of deletions and inversion are similar in their studies from *Nox4*, *Grm5*, and *Nox4-Grm5* (**Table 1**). However, recent results showed the inversion efficiency is lower than deletion in both mice and rats (**Table 1**) [7].

Organism	Mice							
Region of interest	*Tyr* (Exon1-2)	*Tyr*	*Nox4*	*Grm5*	*Nox4-Grm5*	*Hmgn1*	*Tiam1*	*Runx1-Cbr1*
Fragment size	9.4 kb*	65 kb	155 kb	545 kb	1.15 Mb	16.8 kb	226 kb	1.1 Mb
F0-deletion	10%	16%	24%	18%	30%	50%	19.5%	3%***
F0-inversion			30%	18%	21%	0%	0%	3%
F0-duplication			2%	1%	0%	0%	2.4%**	0%***

*Two sgRNAs were used here while all others use four sgRNAs (two 2-sgRNA sets) for the experiments.
**F1 mouse carries duplication detected by droplet digital PCR (ddPCR), although it is not detected in F0 mouse.
***One mouse with duplication and deletion was obtained from a second round of microinjection.

Table 1. Percentage of the rearranged alleles among different loci after CRISPR/Cas9-facilitated chromosome engineering.

3. General CRISPR/Cas9-facilitated chromosome engineering components

The CRISPR/Cas9 system consists of three basic components: (1) CRISPR RNA (crRNA), guiding Cas9 complex to the target sequence; (2) trans-activating crRNA (tracrRNA), hybridizing with crRNA for Cas9 complex targeting; and (3) Cas9 endonuclease, cleaving target double-strand DNA. The damaged DNA will be recognized and repaired in two manners: nonhomologous end joining (NHEJ) and homology-directed repair (HDR) (**Figure 2**) [15, 16]. Besides the aforementioned, there are other considerations that should be noted when designing the CRISPR/Cas9-related experiments, such as the use of bridge sequence, choosing between direct ES cell or zygote injection, and the genotyping strategies through PCR primer designs.

3.1. CRISPR/Cas9 components: guide RNA

To expedite CRISPR/Cas9-facilitated genome manipulation, several groups initially developed a chimeric single guide RNA containing both the crRNA and traccrRNA (sgRNA) [15, 16]. Due to its convenience, the sgRNA has now become the most extensively used RNA template for CRISPR/Cas9-based editing. The sgRNA contains a RNA scaffold with a pre-designed 20 bp RNA sequence, which can bind to the region of interest. Cas9 endonuclease is directed by sgRNA to the targeted sequence and cuts the double-strand DNA. Typically, 10–100 ng/μl of sgRNA has been used in CRISPR/Cas9 system for zygote injection of rodents to generate large structure variations in a genome [7–9].

The number of guide RNA pairs used to target a specific site affects the efficiencies in generating structural variants. It was found by Boroviak et al. [8] that additional double-strand breaks at each endpoint would elevate the frequency of generating structural variants. First, they designed a set of two sgRNAs (2-sgRNA set) for each endpoint that are within 50–200 bp of each other and located on opposite strands of the DNA and then compared the frequency of deletions being generated between different numbers of double-strand breaks (one or two breaks at each endpoint). A 9.4 kb region was cut with two sgRNAs, with one sgRNA at each

http://dx.doi.org/10.5772/intechopen.70897

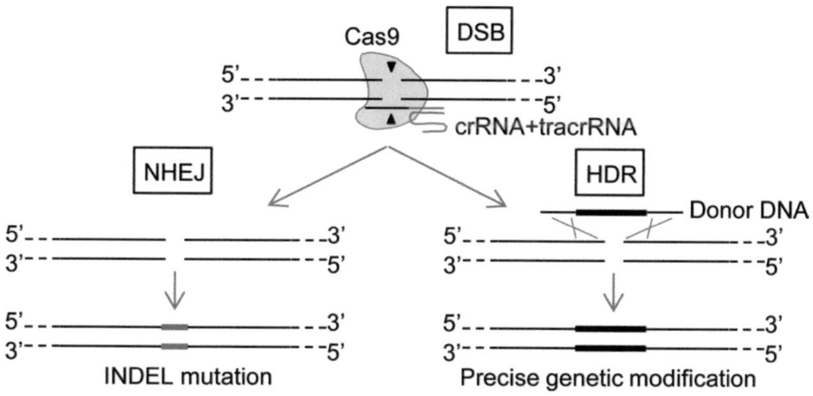

Figure 2. Two types of DNA repairs occur *in vivo* after double-strand breaks caused by Cas9 endonuclease. DSB, double-strand break; crRNA, CRISPR RNA; tracrRNA, trans-activating crRNA; HDR, homology-directed repair; NHEJ, nonhomologous end joining.

endpoint, and the deletion efficiency was found to be 10%, but the frequency of a 65 kb deletion at the same genomic region was increased to 16% when four sgRNAs, with a 2-sgRNA set at each endpoint, were used (see **Table 2**). Boroviak et al. [8] attributed the increase in efficiency to extend the temporal window of DNA breaks before repairing, which provides more opportunities for complete cycles of error-prone repair, and thus resulting in chromosome rearrangement. Birling et al. also believed a 2-sgRNA set at each endpoint would increase the probability of obtaining double-strand breaks [17]. They implemented this strategy to obtain large structural variations in mice and rats using a 2-sgRNA set at each endpoint with a distance of less than 150 bp between the two sgRNAs.

Although sgRNAs have been widely utilized, it is still controversial whether the cleavage efficiency of sgRNA is comparable to those of dual-crRNA:tracrRNA. Unlike sgRNA, in dual-crRNA:tracrRNA, crRNA and tracrRNA are synthesized separately, and then annealed together to be used as the guide RNA [15, 18, 19]. Recently, a few reports have demonstrated that a dual-crRNA:tracrRNA combined with Cas9 protein can increase the efficiency of genome editing, especially the frequency of HDR [18–20]. Therefore, dual-crRNA:tracrRNA should still be considered when planning chromosome rearrangement projects.

Organism	Mice				
Region of interest	*Tyr* (Exon1-2)	*Tyr*	*Nox4*	*Grm5*	*Nox4-Grm5*
Fragment size	9.4 kb*	65 kb	155 kb	545 kb	1.15 Mb
F0-deletion	10%	16%	24%	18%	30%
Imprecise deletion	10%	12%	15%	15%	13%
Precise deletion	0%	4%	9%	3%	17%

*Two sgRNAs were used here while all others use four sgRNAs (two 2-sgRNA sets) for the experiments.

Table 2. Percentage of the precise deletion and imprecise deletion after the introduction of the bridging sequence.

3.2. CRISPR/Cas9 components: Cas9

So far, most of the rodent models with engineered chromosomes have been produced via a one-time injection of Cas9 mRNA and guide RNAs into the zygote cytoplasm. Based on the current literature, 10–200 ng/μl of Cas9 mRNA seems to be sufficient to generate chromosome rearrangements [7, 8]. This approach is both fast and robust, but carries with it the potential complication of genetic mosaicism [21], which may result in different cell populations in F0 founder animals carrying different mutations [8, 22]. For example, up to six different alleles from one single founder have been detected by Birling et al. [17]. Boroviak et al. [8] also showed that many F0 founder mice were genetically mosaic, with up to 4–5 alleles detected. The genetic mosaicism may be due to two possibilities, one being that Cas9 mRNA must first be translated prior to cleavage of the double-strand DNA; however, transcription and translation activity is suppressed in the mouse zygote and de novo translation of Cas9 mRNA might be delayed until second cell stage [21, 23]. The second possibility might be that the functionality of Cas9 and its guide RNA may linger into the 2–4 cell stage and beyond. Likewise, injection of a vast excess of guide RNAs and Cas9 mRNA may result in repeating the cleavage-repair cycles until the targeting site is destroyed by an insertion or deletion (INDEL) or a structural variant [8]. Therefore, zygote injection of Cas9 protein instead of the mRNA may help to reduce mosaicism in founders [21], because Cas9 protein-RNA complex is more likely to degrade rapidly, leading to a shorter half-life than Cas9 mRNA [24–27]. The results from some recent studies support such reasoning [18–20, 26].

3.3. Bridging sequence

Double-strand DNA breaks produced by Cas9 endonuclease are repaired by two major pathways: nonhomologous DNA end joining (NHEJ) and homolog-directed repair (HDR) (**Figure 2**). NHEJ is error-prone and often leads to unpredictable insertions and deletions (INDELs), while HDR introduces precise genetic modification when a template DNA is available [28, 29]. As those unpredictable INDELs might bring out unexpected effects on cells, it is desirable to generate structural variations with nucleotide precision through HDR to repair double-strand DNA breaks. Boroviak et al. [8] established mouse models of deletions with precise endpoints by providing a single strand oligonucleotide DNA as repair template. These oligonucleotides were 120 bp in length and were designed to bridge the deletion juncture. The sequence was designed directly adjacent to the most external guide RNA site but omitting the Cas9 cleavage sites to avoid repeated CRISPR/Cas9 cutting. Boroviak et al. [8] reported a total of 17 out of 53 (32%) deletion mice were born with a precise deletion juncture (**Table 2**).

3.4. Via ES cell manipulation or direct zygote microinjection

Two routes have been used to establish rodent models using CRISPR/Cas9-facilitated chromosome engineering: (1) those produced through transfection of expression vectors containing guide RNAs and Cas9 into embryonic stem cells (ESCs) [9] and (2) models obtained directly from fertilized zygotes injected with guide RNAs and Cas9 mRNA [7, 8].

Kraft et al. [9] introduced the process of using CRISPR/Cas9 technology for generation of structural variations in mouse ESCs. They successfully generated genomic rearrangements across intervals spanning from 1 kb to 1.6 Mb and later showed germline transmission of these rearrangements. Kraft et al. [9] stated that this method for generating structural variations in mice could be accomplished in as short as 10 weeks, yet it is still more time-consuming compared with the method involving direct zygote injection. Boroviak et al. [8] and Birling et al. [7] described their chromosome engineering efforts in mice or rats through cytoplasmic injection of zygotes with Cas9 mRNA and sgRNAs. Both works demonstrated that structural variants of 1 Mb can be efficiently achieved by zygote injection of the CRISPR/Cas9 components. However, the efficiency for generating desired chromosomal duplications appeared less robust when compared to the generation of deletions and inversions. One of the possible reasons is two homologs of the affected chromosome may be involved in generation of a duplication.

3.5. Genotyping strategy for identifying chromosomal structural variations

With these new genetic engineering methods, standard PCR is still primarily the method of choice to identify the structural variants no matter if in ES cell clones or founder mice and rats using CRISPR/Cas9. Since all three types of structural variants, deletion, inversion, and duplication, result in the alteration of the junction region, the approach based on PCR mainly focused on detecting the fragment around the breakpoints in those chromosomes. Selections of appropriate PCR primers are a crucial factor to successfully detect and distinguish different DNA structural variants. The strategy of designing primers is shown in **Table 3**. Usually primers are designed near but outside the areas targeted by guide RNAs or 2 guide RNA sets at each endpoint of the rearrangement fragment. The primer sets near the Cas9 cleavage sites at the head (proximal endpoint closer to the centromere) of the region of interest, forward primer 1 (F1) and reverse primer 1 (R1), and the primer sets at the tail (distal endpoint further from the centromere) of the region of the interest, forward primer 2 (F2), and reverse primer 2 (R2), can be used to identify upstream and downstream double-strand breaks [7]. Different combinations of primers located at proximal and distal ends of the region are required to recognize the structural variation junctions [8]. The combinations are shown in **Table 3**. F1 + R2 primer sets are utilized for deletion analysis, while F1 + F2 and R1 + R2 are for inversion breakpoints. For duplication characterization, different primer sets might be used to distinguish different possibilities. If combining with other primer sets, the direction of the duplication in the genome can be determined. (1) F1 + R1 & F2 + R1 & F2 + R2 could identify the duplication with head-to-tail and head-to-tail orientation as shown in **Table 3**, Dup1. (2) F1 + F2 & R1 + F2 & R1 + R2 primer sets could detect the duplication with tail-to-head and tail-to-head orientation as shown in **Table 3**, Dup2. (3) F1 + F2 & R1 + R1 & F2 + R2 sets could detect the duplication with tail-to-head and head-to-tail orientation as shown in **Table 3**, Dup3. (4) F1 + R1 & F2 + F2 & R1 + R2 sets could detect the duplication with head-to-tail and tail-to-head orientation as shown in **Table 3**, Dup4.

PCR assay is convenient, but it may not be able to reveal extensive information on the chromosome rearrangements. Boroviak et al. [8] reported that in some cases, only one end of the

		PCR primer pairs							
		F1+R1	F2+R2	F1+R2	F1+F2	F2+R1	R1+R2	R1+R1	F2+F2
F1 R1 F2 R2	WT	+	+	-	-	-	-	-	-
F1 R2	Del	-	-	+	-	-	-	-	-
F1 F2 R1 R2	Inv	-	-	-	+	-	+	-	-
F1 R1 F2 R1 F2 R2	Dup1	+	+	-	-	+	-	-	-
F1 F2 R1 F2 R1 R2	Dup2	-	-	-	+	+	+	-	-
F1 F2 R1 R1 F2 R2	Dup3	-	+	-	+	-	-	+	-
F1 R1 F2 F2 R1 R2	Dup4	+	-	-	-	-	+	-	+

Del, deletion; Dup, duplication; F1, forward primer 1; F2, forward primer 2; Inv, inversion; R1, reverse primer 1; R2, reverse primer 2.

Table 3. PCR strategies for identifying the rearranged alleles after CRISPR/Cas9-facilitated recombination.

inversion could be detected rather than two ends. Birling et al. [17] also mentioned that deletion of *Dyrk1a* region in rats cannot be detected by standard PCR, but they discovered 4 founder rats carried one copy of *Dyrk1a* gene through droplet digital PCR (ddPCR). These false negative results indicated the junction areas may be changed during DNA cleavage and repair; therefore, it stops the primer from binding to the expected site. Thus, other approaches need to be considered to complement standard PCR for identifying structural variations when using CRIPSR/Cas9 system. For example, ddPCR and real-time PCR can be utilized for determining copy number variants in genome.

4. Summary

With the addition of the techniques of CRISPR/Cas9-facilitated chromosome engineering beyond the current tools, it is reasonable to predict that many important insights of DS will be revealed in the near future, which will surely be a welcome news since they may be instrumental for developing next therapeutic strategies for this important genetic disorder.

Acknowledgements

The projects in Eugene Yu's laboratory were supported in part by grants from Roswell Park Alliance Foundation, the Children's Guild Foundation, the NIH (R01HL91519, R01NS66072, R21GM114645, and P30CA16056).

Author details

Zhuo Xing[1], Yichen Li[1], Annie Pao[1], Garrett Kaas[2] and Y. Eugene Yu[1,3]*

*Address all correspondence to: yuejin.yu@roswellpark.org

1 Department of Cancer Genetics and Genomics, Roswell Park Cancer Institute, Buffalo, NY, USA

2 Department of Pharmacology, Vanderbilt University, Nashville, Tennessee, USA

3 State University of New York at Buffalo, Buffalo, NY, USA

References

[1] Davisson MT, Schmidt C, Akeson EC. Segmental trisomy of murine chromosome 16: A new model system for studying Down syndrome. Progress in Clinical and Biological Research. 1990;**360**:263-280

[2] O'Doherty A, Ruf S, Mulligan C, Hildreth V, Errington ML, et al. An aneuploid mouse strain carrying human chromosome 21 with Down syndrome phenotypes. Science. 2005; **309**:2033-2037

[3] Gribble SM, Wiseman FK, Clayton S, Prigmore E, Langley E, et al. Massively parallel sequencing reveals the complex structure of an irradiated human chromosome on a mouse background in the Tc1 model of Down syndrome. PLoS One. 2013;**8**:e60482

[4] Yu T, Li Z, Jia Z, Clapcote SJ, Liu C, et al. A mouse model of Down syndrome trisomic for all human chromosome 21 syntenic regions. Human Molecular Genetics. 2010; **19**:2780-2791

[5] Herault Y, Delabar J, Fisher EMC, Tybulewicz VLJ, Yu E, et al. Rodents models in Down syndrome research: Impact and future opportunities. Disease Models & Mechanisms. 2017;**10**:1165-1186

[6] Xing Z, Li Y, Pao A, Bennett AS, Tycko B, et al. Mouse-based genetic modeling and analysis of Down syndrome. British Medical Bulletin. 2016;**120**:111-122

[7] Birling MC, Schaeffer L, Andre P, Lindner L, Marechal D, et al. Efficient and rapid generation of large genomic variants in rats and mice using CRISMERE. Scientific Reports. 2017;**7**:43331

[8] Boroviak K, Doe B, Banerjee R, Yang F, Bradley A. Chromosome engineering in zygotes with CRISPR/Cas9. Genesis. 2016;**54**:78-85

[9] Kraft K, Geuer S, Will AJ, Chan WL, Paliou C, et al. Deletions, inversions, duplications: Engineering of structural variants using CRISPR/Cas in mice. Cell Reports. 2015

[10] Lagutina IV, Valentine V, Picchione F, Harwood F, Valentine MB, et al. Modeling of the human alveolar rhabdomyosarcoma Pax3-Foxo1 chromosome translocation in mouse myoblasts using CRISPR-Cas9 nuclease. PLoS Genetics. 2015;**11**:e1004951

[11] Yu Y, Bradley A. Engineering chromosomal rearrangements in mice. Nature Reviews. Genetics. 2001;**2**:780-790

[12] Niu Y, Shen B, Cui Y, Chen Y, Wang J, et al. Generation of gene-modified cynomolgus monkey via Cas9/RNA-mediated gene targeting in one-cell embryos. Cell. 2014; **156**:836-843

[13] Wang H, Yang H, Shivalila CS, Dawlaty MM, Cheng AW, et al. One-step generation of mice carrying mutations in multiple genes by CRISPR/Cas-mediated genome engineering. Cell. 2013;**153**:910-918

[14] Yang H, Wang H, Shivalila CS, Cheng AW, Shi L, et al. One-step generation of mice carrying reporter and conditional alleles by CRISPR/Cas-mediated genome engineering. Cell. 2013;**154**:1370-1379

[15] Cong L, Ran FA, Cox D, Lin S, Barretto R, et al. Multiplex genome engineering using CRISPR/Cas systems. Science. 2013;**339**:819-823

[16] Jinek M, Chylinski K, Fonfara I, Hauer M, Doudna JA, et al. A programmable dual-RNA-guided DNA endonuclease in adaptive bacterial immunity. Science. 2012;**337**:816-821

[17] Birling MC, Herault Y, Pavlovic G. Modeling human disease in rodents by CRISPR/Cas9 genome editing. Mammalian Genome. 2017;**28**:291-301

[18] Aida T, Chiyo K, Usami T, Ishikubo H, Imahashi R, et al. Cloning-free CRISPR/Cas system facilitates functional cassette knock-in in mice. Genome Biology. 2015;**16**:87

[19] Quadros RM, Miura H, Harms DW, Akatsuka H, Sato T, et al. Easi-CRISPR: A robust method for one-step generation of mice carrying conditional and insertion alleles using long ssDNA donors and CRISPR ribonucleoproteins. Genome Biology. 2017;**18**:92

[20] Chen S, Lee B, Lee AY, Modzelewski AJ, He L. Highly efficient mouse genome editing by CRISPR ribonucleoprotein electroporation of zygotes. The Journal of Biological Chemistry. 2016;**291**:14457-14467

[21] Hsu PD, Lander ES, Zhang F. Development and applications of CRISPR-Cas9 for genome engineering. Cell. 2014;**157**:1262-1278

[22] Yen ST, Zhang M, Deng JM, Usman SJ, Smith CN, et al. Somatic mosaicism and allele complexity induced by CRISPR/Cas9 RNA injections in mouse zygotes. Developmental Biology. 2014;**393**:3-9

[23] Oh B, Hwang S, McLaughlin J, Solter D, Knowles BB. Timely translation during the mouse oocyte-to-embryo transition. Development. 2000;**127**:3795-3803

[24] Kim S, Kim D, Cho SW, Kim J, Kim JS. Highly efficient RNA-guided genome editing in human cells via delivery of purified Cas9 ribonucleoproteins. Genome Research. 2014;**24**:1012-1019

[25] Lin S, Staahl BT, Alla RK, Doudna JA. Enhanced homology-directed human genome engineering by controlled timing of CRISPR/Cas9 delivery. eLife. 2014;**3**:e04766

[26] Ma X, Chen C, Veevers J, Zhou X, Ross RS, et al. CRISPR/Cas9-mediated gene manipulation to create single-amino-acid-substituted and floxed mice with a cloning-free method. Scientific Reports. 2017;**7**:42244

[27] Ramakrishna S, Kwaku Dad AB, Beloor J, Gopalappa R, Lee SK, et al. Gene disruption by cell-penetrating peptide-mediated delivery of Cas9 protein and guide RNA. Genome Research. 2014;**24**:1020-1027

[28] Chu VT, Weber T, Wefers B, Wurst W, Sander S, et al. Increasing the efficiency of homology-directed repair for CRISPR-Cas9-induced precise gene editing in mammalian cells. Nature Biotechnology. 2015;**33**:543-548

[29] Maruyama T, Dougan SK, Truttmann MC, Bilate AM, Ingram JR, et al. Increasing the efficiency of precise genome editing with CRISPR-Cas9 by inhibition of nonhomologous end joining. Nature Biotechnology. 2015;**33**:538-542

Section 2

Mental Retardation and Cognitive Disability

Chapter 2

Psychopathology in Down Syndrome

Sevde Afife Ersoy, Hasan Ali Güler and
Fatih Hilmi Çetin

Additional information is available at the end of the chapter

http://dx.doi.org/10.5772/intechopen.71061

Abstract

The main aim of this section is to provide clinicians with a guide to the prevalence of psychopathologies, associated factors, and their treatment in children with Down syndrome (DS). Attention-deficit/hyperactivity disorder (ADHD), behavioral disorders, depression, and autism are more common in DS than the normal population. However, the incidence of psychopathology is generally lower in DS than in other diseases that cause mental retardation. While writing this chapter, approximately 200 articles in electronic databases were scanned using the keywords "Down Syndrome and Psychopathology," "Down Syndrome and Mood Disorder," "Down Syndrome and Autism," "Down Syndrome and Anxiety," "Down Syndrome and Catatonia," and "Down Syndrome and Behavioral Disorder." Psychopathologies in DS will be presented in eight subtitles beginning with the most often diagnosed. It is important to perform psychological evaluations of patients with DS during routine follow-ups. Comorbid diseases (obstructive sleep apnea, cardiac pathologies, etc.) should be taken into account when choosing drugs.

Keywords: down syndrome, psychopathology, mental health

1. Introduction

Down syndrome (DS) is the most common chromosomal anomaly which is associated with intellectual disability (ID), typical physical features, and health problems. The incidence of DS is about 1–1.5 of every 1000 live births. DS is the most frequent genetic cause of mental retardation (MR) [1]. People with MR have behavioral, emotional, and psychiatric problems more often than the general population [2].

DS exhibits distinctive neurodevelopmental, neurocognitive, and psychopathological patterns when compared to other genetic syndromes leading to ID, albeit higher than the general population [3]. A 28.9% of the children with DS have psychiatric comorbidity [4]. The children with DS are more likely to have externalizing behaviors than their siblings and peers, including hyperactivity, impulsivity, inattention, tantrums, agitation, stubbornness, disruptiveness/argumentativeness, oppositionality, repetitive movements, sensory dysregulation, and speech problems despite being recognized as friendly, easygoing, good tempered, affectionate, and sympathetic individuals [3, 5, 6]. The rate of severe behavior disorder in children with DS is reported as 23% [7]. The 4- to 18-year-old children with DS are more likely to exhibit such externalizing behaviors compared to normal-developing controls; 6–8% of children with DS are diagnosed with attention-deficit/hyperactivity disorder (ADHD); and 10–15% of children or youth are diagnosed with behavioral or oppositional disorders [2]. Externalizing behaviors change into internalizing behaviors in adolescents with DS. Internalizing behavior problems such as withdrawal, shyness, low confidence, and depression are more common in adolescents and adults [2]. A longitudinal cohort study showed that the incidence of depressive disorders was 5.2% of the total sample of adolescents and adults (16 years) with DS [8]. Depressive symptoms can also be seen with increased maladaptive behaviors other than known symptoms deteriorating speech and adaptive skills and fluctuating motor symptoms. As in the general population, anxiety symptoms such as fear, trembling, flushing, and irritability can be observed in DS [9]. However, there is not enough data on the incidence and prevalence of anxiety symptoms in DS. Some have shown that the prevalence of obsessive-compulsive disorder (OCD) in DS ranges from 0.8 to 4.5% and not much higher than the general population. These rates may be low because it is difficult to assess the obsessions and compulsions in individuals with cognitive impairment. As for OCD, there is a lower prevalence of schizophrenia and bipolar disorder in individuals with DS [3]. In latest studies, the co-occurrence of DS and autism spectrum disorders (ASD) has increased ratio; approximately 6–10% of children have comorbid ASD [5]. Compared with the children with ASD in general, the children with DS are diagnosed with ASD in 6–16 years of age. The syndrome that may overlap with DS phenotypic social communication patterns may be difficult to define in the DS population due to behavioral diagnostic criteria [10].

The prevalence of DS was 5.9 per 10,000 general population. Point prevalence of mental disorder of any type varied from 23.7 to 10.8%; 2-year incidence varied from 14.9 to 3.7% [8]. This suggests that psychopathology is not seen in a minor proportion of individuals with DS. In this article, we aimed to define psychopathology in individuals with DS and to guide the clinicians in diagnosis and treatment.

2. Attention-deficit/hyperactivity disorder (ADHD)

ADHD is a developmental disorder with a prevalence of 5% in the community [11]. ADHD frequency in DS is 14–43.9% [12, 13].

It was thought that attention deficit and hyperactivity are caused by maturation retardation in the past years, and therefore there should not be an additional diagnosis other than mental retardation [14]. Diagnostic overshadowing has been used to describe this situation [15]. However, according to both the Diagnostic and Statistical Manual of Mental Disorders-IV (DSM-IV) and the DSM-V, mental retardation is not an exclusion criterion for ADHD [16, 17].

ADHD has three main symptoms: inattention, impulsivity, and hyperactivity, which are disproportionate to mental age. These symptoms can be observed in children with DS, but impulsivity and hyperactivity are more prominent up to 36 months [18]. In a study in 14 DS children (aged 2–4 years), ADHD was diagnosed in 30% of the children [19].

The children with DS may have mental retardation in mild (IQ 50–70), moderate (IQ 35–50), or severe (IQ 20–35) levels [20]. Studies of whether there is a correlation between the symptoms of ADHD and the degree of mental retardation are contradictory [12, 19, 21, 22]. It is known that executive functions are inadequate in ADHD. DS is also known to be inadequate in executive functions (especially in process memory) [23, 24]. Visual and hearing loss, obstructive sleep apnea, and thyroid disease associated with DS may mimic symptoms of ADHD [12].

The most commonly used drugs in the treatment of ADHD are psychostimulants and atomoxetine. Psychostimulants are the first line of treatment [25–28]. However, cardiac pathology in 50% of DS patients lead to the preference of other drug groups such as alpha-adrenergic agonists in place of methylphenidate in the treatment of ADHD [29, 30]. In addition, the presence of decreased dopamine beta-hydroxylase and increased catechol-o-methyltransferase activity in DS also modifies methylphenidate efficacy [31]. In support of this view, the only study of ADHD treatment in DS was performed using guanfacine. Twenty-three children aged between 4 and 12 years were included in the study and given guanfacine treatment. The effect size of guanfacine for inattention was found to be 0.7, and the effect size for hyperactivity was found to be 0.9; no serious side effects were reported [18]. Thus, there is a need for more research for the treatment of ADHD in DS.

3. Conduct disorder

Conduct disorder as other psychopathologies is more common in children with mental retardation [32]. More than 10% of the children with DS were diagnosed with conduct disorder [33]. Conduct disorder prevalence in DS is lower than other pathologies causing mental retardation [34].

Externalizing behaviors in DS is more common than internalizing behavior [35]. In a study, which used the Child Behavior Checklist and included 211 children with DS, stubbornness (79%) and disobedience (74%) were reported. Stubbornness has been reported to be a characteristic of DS. In the same study, behavioral problems peaked between 10 and 13 years of age, and in accordance with clinical practice, externalizing behavior was reduced toward late adolescence and internalizing behavior was increased. However, in both adult and pediatric samples, it has been found that fighting (12%) and excessive physical aggression (6%) in individuals with DS are rare [36].

Some atypical antipsychotics approved by the Food and Drug Administration (FDA) for the treatment of aggression in autism are often used off-label in the treatment of aggression in patients with mental retardation [37]. Studies have shown that the use of atypical antipsychotics in DS peaked between 11 and 14 years of age. This age range is also the period when behavior problems are frequently seen in DS. Behavioral problems in DS are more common in males than in females, and consistent with this, atypical antipsychotic use is more common in males [28, 36]. Thus, there is a need for new studies, especially on drug treatment.

4. Depression

The prevalence of psychopathology is higher in DS than healthy population [34]. However, psychopathology is less frequent in DS compared to other children with intellectual disability [3]. The prevalence of depression in DS is 11%; DS is also a risk factor for developing depression [38, 39]. Depression frequency is lower in children and adolescents with DS than adults [40].

Stress-related disorders, such as depression, are the result of complex interactions of external stressors and biological factors [41]. Cognitive impairment and inadequacy of problem-solving skills lead to social rejection and failure [42]. In DS, the total brain volume and hippocampus volume are smaller than the normal population, leading to an increased risk of depression [43, 44]. These structural changes in the brain are thought to be caused by a protein overexpression encoded on chromosome 21 [45]. It is thought that serotonin, an important neurotransmitter in brain development, is deficient in fetal life in individuals with DS and that this deficiency continues in adulthood and increases susceptibility to depression [46].

Diagnosing depression is difficult in children with DS due to various problems related to neurophysiological developments (retardation in nonverbal communication, delay in speech) [28]. The most common symptom of depression in DS is the loss of interest (95.4%). In addition, changes in sleep and appetite patterns (81.8%), agitation (72%), and anxiety (40.9%) are other common symptoms [47]. Suicidal thoughts and guilt are rare [48].

In a study, only half of the 56 patients with DS who were diagnosed with depression were found to meet the criteria for major depression according to the Diagnostic and Statistical Manual of Mental Disorders. This is thought to be due to the lack of separate diagnostic criteria for patients with mental retardation [49].

Depression in people with DS needs to be separated from hypothyroidism, because hypothyroidism is more common among people with DS than the normal population [50]. In addition, sleep apnea, which may mimic depression, may be diagnosed at a rate of 30–60% in DS [39, 51].

The most commonly used drug is selective serotonin reuptake inhibitors (SSRI), but there is no controlled study in this respect [52]. In a retrospective study involving 832 children and adolescents with DS, the rate of SSRI use was 9.6% for 5- to 11-year olds and 7.6% for 12- to 21-year olds [28]. In a study compiling case reports, antidepressant treatment response rate was found to be 50% [49]. In addition, electroconvulsive therapy and psychotherapies can be used in therapy [53–55].

5. Autism

Autism spectrum disorder (ASD) is a neurodevelopmental disorder characterized by restricted, repetitive behavior and interests and difficulties in social communication and social interaction. The prevalence of autism in the world is about 1%, and approximately 45% of the cases are accompanied by intellectual disability. About 5–39% of ASD individuals have DS and 1–11% of DS individuals have ASD. Autism is more common among individuals with DS than the general population [56, 57].

ASD was reported in other chromosome abnormalities (21–50% of affected individuals have autism in fragile X syndrome, 24–60% in tuberous sclerosis complex, 50–81% in Angelman syndrome, 60–70% in Timothy syndrome, ~40% in Joubert syndrome, 5–20% in phenylketonuria, and 15–50% in CHARGE syndrome). DS is a chromosomal anomaly characterized by trisomy 21. Overlapping or co-occurrence of DS and ASD mechanisms is uncertain. Obstetric difficulties and/or fetal maldevelopment, congenital or early-acquired brain defects, vulnerability to anoxia, infection, or other harmful effects during the intrauterine or neonatal period as a result of chromosome abnormalities are some of the etiological factors suggested for DS and ASD in literature. Hereditary factors, epilepsy, and hypothyroidism are other medical conditions likely to cause autism in DS [13, 56, 58].

Meta-analyses and postmortem studies suggest that both autism and DS have neuropathological features in cerebellar and cerebral cortices such as heterotopic areas or focal abnormal gray matter density differences (amygdala, hippocampus, temporal lobe, cerebellum). These neuroanatomical differences, although not specific to autism and DS, may reflect changing functional organization patterns that are common to both [3, 56]. Cerebellum and brainstem white matters have increased volumes in individuals with autism along with DS in comparison to those without autism. These areas associated with stereotypes [59].

The children with DS are diagnosed with ASD in 6–16 years of age compared to the children with ASD only. The disorder, which may overlap with the phenotypic social communication patterns of DS, may be difficult to define in the DS population because the behavioral diagnostic criteria and regression occur later; an onset between 3 and 8 years of age may also be a reason for the delay in diagnosis [10, 57].

DS individuals without autism are communicated and socially motivated despite their verbal disabilities and show more advanced interpersonal relationships and play and leisure time skills than children with ASD. The evidence of autism are impairment of communicative gesture, mime, and facial expression; impairment in the ability to initiate or sustain conversation; social reciprocity; lack of eye contact; poor social orienting; infrequent social overtures; poor integration of verbal and nonverbal behaviors; lack of joint attention; restricted shared effect; inconsistent social responding (tendency to be alone, difficulty in interacting with children); constrained imitation; failure to develop functional means of communication; delayed speech (although motor milestones such as sitting and walking without support are within normal limits); habit of making irrelevant remarks; repeating the other person's phrases; echolalia; dull and repetitive play (such as rolling a toy over and over again); repetitive movements (such as frequent tapping of feet, flapping of arms, constant rocking of the body, compulsive touching of people, indiscriminate habit of feeling the texture of objects); undue attachment to certain objects; and distress over changes in environment [60, 61]. All these evidence are might also be seen DS individuals with autism. Individuals with DS alone may show language stereotypes, specific interests in parts of objects, rituals, specific body use, and strange behavioral patterns specific to DS. ASD in DS is diagnosed with specific autistic features that include phenotypic behavioral features which may be determined by through and widely used screening tools (ADOS, CARS, M-CHAT) and DSM-V criteria [57].

The treatment and monitoring program should be structured according to the functional level and the disability areas of the affected person because each individual with DS has problems at different levels. Treatment approaches in ASD can be grouped into two categories as "educational treatments" and "pharmacological treatments."

There is no medical agent for treating the core symptoms of autism. But antipsychotic drugs (haloperidol, risperidone, aripiprazole) have been shown to effectively reduce challenging, stereotypic behaviors, irritability, tantrum, and hyperactivity. Educational approaches are the most effective approach to alleviate basic symptoms and increase functioning in autism [62, 63].

Early diagnosis of ASD in DS is important so that convenient educational, behavioral, rehabilitative, and therapeutic interventions and strategies are available to help ensure that children receive the best possible outcomes.

6. Obsessive-compulsive disorder (OCD)

Obsessive-compulsive disorder (OCD) is characterized by the presence of obsessions and compulsions. Obsessions are thought, impulse, and dreams in which attempts to disengage, if accepted as repetitive, disturbing, and illogical, have failed. Compulsions are repetitive behaviors and mental actions that appear to reduce obsessions and reduce anxiety caused by obsessions. OCD was classified with DSM-5 under the heading "Obsessive-Compulsive and Related Disorders" by subtracting it from the heading of "Anxiety Disorders" [64].

The prevalence of OCD in a follow-up study was reported as 3.5% [65], and other studies have shown that the prevalence of OCD among individuals with DS ranges from 0.8 to 4.5% and not much higher than the general population. These rates may be low because it is difficult to assess the obsessions and compulsions in individuals with cognitive impairment. OCD increases similar to depression and other internalizing behavior problems among adolescents and adults with DS.

The individuals with DS present with ordering and tidiness compulsions, which are the most commonly reported OCD symptoms. On the other hand "obsessional slowness" is described as a ritualistic behavior that is the part of compulsion in individuals with DS. In case reports, OCD symptoms such as compulsively turning off lights, insisting that all doors needed to be shut, aligning the objects like books and pictures, hoarding behaviors such as keeping objects (water bottles, sunglasses, and boxes), touching rituals (touching the floor in a ritualistic manner several times, touching each of clothes hangers routinely each morning), fastidiousness, spend excessive amounts of time in the bathroom, taking too long to complete daily routine (slowness in daily living skills, eating, and walking), perfectionism, and checking were reported.

The first line of pharmacological treatment for OCD includes SSRIs. Switching to another SSRI, augmentation with neuroleptics and the use of a serotonin norepinephrine agent are suggested as pharmacological treatment options for treatment-resistant OCD [66]. In literature, it was shown that SSRIs were effective with OCD in DS, and neuroleptic augmentation was effective with treatment-resistant OCD in DS. Also, recent studies suggest that glutamatergic agents such as memantine are effective in treatment-resistant OCD in both individuals with or without DS [67].

7. Anxiety disorders

Fear and anxiety are necessary to survive by resisting danger and threat. Although it is an adaptive process, fear and anxiety may become pathological when they are incited by objects or situations that are not legitimately harmful or threatening and restrict the person's functioning [68]. Anxiety disorders include specific phobias, separation anxiety disorder, selective mutism, social anxiety disorder (social phobia), generalized anxiety disorder, panic disorder, panic attack specifier and agoraphobia, substance-/medication-induced anxiety disorder, anxiety disorder due to another medical condition, other specified anxiety disorders, and unspecified anxiety disorder [16].

DS exhibits distinctive neurodevelopmental, neurocognitive, and psychopathological patterns when compared to other genetic syndromes leading to ID, albeit higher than the general population [3]. People with ID often have more behavioral, emotional, and psychiatric problems than the general population [2]. Anxiety disorder is one of these psychiatric problems. Studies suggest that 10–22% of the individuals with ID have met diagnostic criteria for anxiety disorder; this rate is higher than the individuals with typical development (3–7%). Studies have found no difference in prevalence of anxiety among mentally disabled individuals between the genders [69]. As in the general population, anxiety symptoms such as fear, trembling, flushing, and irritability can be observed in DS [9]. However, there is no enough data on the incidence and prevalence of anxiety symptoms in DS.

Children with DS are more common to have externalizing behaviors than their siblings and peers despite being recognized as friendly, easygoing, good tempered, affectionate, and sympathetic individuals; these behaviors include hyperactivity, impulsivity, inattention, tantrums, agitation, stubbornness, disruptiveness/argumentativeness, oppositionality, repetitive movements, sensory dysregulation, and speech problems [3, 5, 6]. ADHD and anxiety comorbidities were found higher among individuals with DS-ID than in typically developed individuals [3, 69].

Treatment of anxiety disorders in childhood contains psychotherapeutic and psychopharmacological interventions, specifically cognitive behavioral therapy (CBT), behavioral therapy, and SSRIs. However, there is no enough study in literature for anxiety in DS and treatment of anxiety in DS [68]. There is a need for more studies on this subject.

8. Bipolar disorder

There is no study on the prevalence of bipolar disorder in children and adolescents, but the prevalence of bipolar disorder is 1% in life. Interestingly, it was found to be 0.3% in DS. This rate is 1.6% in other disorders causing mental retardation. Bipolar disorder in DS is less common than the normal population, leading to the hypothesis that the susceptibility to bipolar disorder may be on chromosome 21. Recent studies have also shown that the susceptibility to bipolar disorder is in the 21q22 locus, which expresses the protein that regulates intracellular calcium concentration [70, 71]. Thus, individuals with DS with an extra chromosome 21 can compensate for the potential effects of the chromosome 21 with the disease [72].

9. Catatonia

Catatonia is a neuropsychiatric syndrome with typical motor indications and responds to electroconvulsive therapy and benzodiazepines [73]. The main signs are changes in motor activity, movement disorders (stereotype, grimas, and tics), changes in speech, impairment of oral intake, negativism, and urinary and gaita incontinence [74]. Neurological, autoimmune, and infectious causes must be excluded before the diagnosis of catatonia [75].

The prevalence of catatonia among children and adolescents with DS is not fully known, but case reports are available in the literature. In four case reports published in 2015, patients who were diagnosed with catatonia and did not respond to benzodiazepine treatment were treated with electroconvulsive therapy [48, 75].

The clinician should examine catatonia when regression—sudden loss of good acquired skills—is present. A significant number of adolescents with DS experience regression. In such a case, comprehensive psychiatric and physical examination is required for diagnosis. Physical examination is especially important for the exclusion of autoimmune and neurological diseases. A dramatic response to 1–2 mg lorazepam administration is a typical sign in catatonia. Symptoms such as mood swings, loss of interest and desire, and sleep and appetite disorders that can be seen in mood disorders can also be seen in the catatonia. The motor symptoms seen in the catatonia and the inability to respond to antidepressant and mood stabilizers in treatment are used in differential diagnosis. Individuals with DS generally do not respond to benzodiazepine therapy and require electroconvulsive therapy [27, 75, 76].

In conclusion, studies suggest that children with DS are at increased risk of having psychopathologies. The clinicians should not neglect the psychopathology in DS and must direct DS individuals to psychiatric examination and treatment. Nevertheless, there is a need for further studies about DS and psychopathology.

Author details

Sevde Afife Ersoy, Hasan Ali Güler and Fatih Hilmi Çetin*

*Address all correspondence to: fatihhilmicetin@gmail.com

Selçuk University Faculty of Medicine, Child of Adolescent Psychiatry Department, Konya, Turkey

References

[1] Cocchi G, Gualdi S, Bower C, Halliday J, Jonsson B, Myrelid Å, et al. International trends of down syndrome 1993-2004: Births in relation to maternal age and terminations of pregnancies. Birth Defects Research Part A: Clinical and Molecular Teratology. 2010;**88**(6):474-479

[2] Dykens EM. Psychiatric and behavioral disorders in persons with down syndrome. Developmental Disabilities Research Reviews. 2007;**13**(3):272-278

[3] Vicari S, Pontillo M, Armando M. Neurodevelopmental and psychiatric issues in Down's syndrome: Assessment and intervention. Psychiatric Genetics. 2013;**23**(3):95-107

[4] Prasher V, Day S. Brief report: Obsessive-compulsive disorder in adults with Down's syndrome. Journal of Autism and Developmental Disorders. 1995;**25**(4):453-458

[5] Grieco J, Pulsifer M, Seligsohn K, Skotko B, Schwartz A, editors. Down Syndrome: Cognitive and Behavioral Functioning across the Lifespan. American Journal of Medical Genetics Part C: Seminars in Medical Genetics. 2015;**169**(2):135-149

[6] Gau SS-F, Chiu Y-N, Soong W-T, Lee M-B. Parental characteristics, parenting style, and behavioral problems among Chinese children with down syndrome, their siblings and controls in Taiwan. Journal of the Formosan Medical Association. 2008;**107**(9):693-703

[7] McCarthy J. Behaviour problems and adults with down syndrome: Childhood risk factors. Journal of Intellectual Disability Research. 2008;**52**(10):877-882

[8] Mantry D, Cooper SA, Smiley E, Morrison J, Allan L, Williamson A, et al. The prevalence and incidence of mental ill-health in adults with down syndrome. Journal of Intellectual Disability Research. 2008;**52**(2):141-155

[9] Fletcher R, Loschen E, Stavrakaki C, et al., editors. Diagnostic Manual-Intellectual Disability: A Textbook of Diagnosis of Mental Disorders in Persons with Intellectual Disability. Kingston, NY: NADD, 2007

[10] Reilly C. Autism spectrum disorders in down syndrome: A review. Research in Autism Spectrum Disorders. 2009;**3**(4):829-839

[11] Banaschewski T, Becker K, Döpfner M, Holtmann M, Rösler M, Romanos M. Attention-deficit/hyperactivity disorder. Deutsches Arzteblatt International. 2017;**114**(9):149-159

[12] Ekstein S, Glick B, Weill M, Kay B, Berger I. Down syndrome and attention-deficit/hyperactivity disorder (ADHD). Journal of Child Neurology. 2011;**26**(10):1290-1295

[13] Oxelgren UW, Myrelid Å, Annerén G, Ekstam B, Göransson C, Holmbom A, et al. Prevalence of autism and attention-deficit–hyperactivity disorder in Down syndrome: A population-based study. Developmental Medicine & Child Neurology. 2017;**59**(3):276-283

[14] Hastings RP, Beck A, Daley D, Hill C. Symptoms of ADHD and their correlates in children with intellectual disabilities. Research in Developmental Disabilities. 2005;**26**(5):456-468

[15] Reiss S, Levitan GW, Szyszko J. Emotional disturbance and mental retardation: Diagnostic overshadowing. American Journal of Mental Deficiency. 1982

[16] Association AP. Diagnostic and Statistical Manual of Mental Disorders (DSM-5®). American Psychiatric Pub, Arlington-USA. 2013

[17] Association AP. Diagnostic and Statistical Manual of Mental Disorders, Text Revision (DSM-IV-TR). Washington, DC: American Psychiatric Publishing; 2000

[18] Capone GT, Brecher L, Bay M. Guanfacine use in children with down syndrome and comorbid attention-deficit hyperactivity disorder (ADHD) with disruptive behaviors. Journal of Child Neurology. 2016;**31**(8):957-964

[19] Green JM, Dennis J, Bennets L. Attention disorder in a group of young Down's syndrome children. Journal of Intellectual Disability Research. 1989;**33**(2):105-122

[20] Cunniff C, Frias JL, Kaye C, Moeschler JB, Panny SR, Trotter TL, et al. Health supervision for children with down syndrome. Pediatrics. 2001;**107**(2):442-449

[21] Fidan T, Kirpinar I, Oral M, Koçak K. Is there a relationship between attention deficit/hyperactivity disorder and manic symptoms among children with mental retardation of unknown etiology? Comprehensive Psychiatry. 2011;**52**(6):644-649

[22] Nærland T, Bakke K, Storvik S, Warner G, Howlin P. Age and gender-related differences in emotional and behavioural problems and autistic features in children and adolescents with down syndrome: A survey-based study of 674 individuals. Journal of Intellectual Disability Research. 2017;**61**(6):594-603

[23] Doyle AE. Executive functions in attention-deficit/hyperactivity disorder. The Journal of Clinical Psychiatry. 2006;**67**:21-26

[24] Loveall S, Conners F, Tungate A, Hahn L, Osso T. A cross-sectional analysis of executive function in down syndrome from 2 to 35 years. Journal of Intellectual Disability Research. 2017;**61**(9):877-887

[25] Pliszka S, Issues AWGQ. Practice parameter for the assessment and treatment of children and adolescents with attention-deficit/hyperactivity disorder. Journal of the American Academy of Child & Adolescent Psychiatry. 2007;**46**(7):894-921

[26] Çuhadaroğlu Çetin F, Coşkun A, İşeri E. Çocuk ve ergen psikiyatrisi temel kitabı. 1. Ankara: Baskı Hekimler Yayın Birliği; 2008. p. 647-660

[27] Stein DS, Munir KM, Karweck AJ, Davidson EJ, Stein MT. Developmental regression, depression, and psychosocial stress in an adolescent with Down syndrome. Journal of Developmental and Behavioral Pediatrics: JDBP. 2013;**34**(3):216-218

[28] Downes A, Anixt JS, Esbensen AJ, Wiley S, Meinzen-Derr J. Psychotropic medication use in children and adolescents with down syndrome. Journal of Developmental & Behavioral Pediatrics. 2015;**36**(8):613-619

[29] Roizen NJ, Patterson D. Down's syndrome. The Lancet. 2003;**361**(9365):1281-1289

[30] Subcommittee on attention-deficit/hyperactivity disorder, steering committee on quality improvement and management. ADHD: clinical practice guideline for the diagnosis, evaluation, and treatment of attention-deficit/hyperactivity disorder in children and adolescents. Pediatrics. 2011;**128**(5):1007-1022

[31] Coyle JT, Oster-Granite M, Gearhart JD. The neurobiologie consequences of down syndrome. Brain Research Bulletin. 1986;**16**(6):773-787

[32] Emerson E. Prevalence of psychiatric disorders in children and adolescents with and without intellectual disability. Journal of Intellectual Disability Research. 2003;**47**(1):51-58

[33] Coe DA, Matson JL, Russell DW, Slifer KJ, Capone GT, Baglio C, et al. Behavior problems of children with down syndrome and life events. Journal of Autism and Developmental Disorders. 1999;**29**(2):149-156

[34] Collacott RA, Cooper S-A, McGROTHER C. Differential rates of psychiatric disorders in adults with Down's syndrome compared with other mentally handicapped adults. The British Journal of Psychiatry. 1992;**161**(5):671-674

[35] Dykens EM, Kasari C. Maladaptive behavior in children with Prader-Willi syndrome, down syndrome, and nonspecific mental retardation. American Journal on Mental Retardation. 1997;**102**(3):228-237

[36] Dykens EM, Shah B, Sagun J, Beck T, King B. Maladaptive behaviour in children and adolescents with Down's syndrome. Journal of Intellectual Disability Research. 2002;**46**(6):484-492

[37] Harrison JN, Cluxton-Keller F, Gross D. Antipsychotic medication prescribing trends in children and adolescents. Journal of Pediatric Health Care. 2012;**26**(2):139-145

[38] McGuire D, Chicoine B. Depressive disorders in adults with down syndrome. Habilitative mental healthcare. Newsletter. 1996;**15**(1):26-27

[39] Capone G, Goyal P, Ares W, Lannigan E, editors. Neurobehavioral disorders in children, adolescents, and young adults with Down syndrome. American Journal of Medical Genetics Part C: Seminars in Medical Genetics. 2006;**142**C:158-172

[40] Määttä T, Tervo-Määttä T, Taanila A, Kaski M, Iivanainen M. Mental health, behaviour and intellectual abilities of people with down syndrome. Down Syndrome Research and Practice. 2006;**11**(1):37-43

[41] Monroe SM, Simons AD. Diathesis-stress theories in the context of life stress research: Implications for the depressive disorders. Psychological Bulletin. 1991;**110**(3):406

[42] Cooper S-A, Smiley E, Morrison J, Williamson A, Allan L. An epidemiological investigation of affective disorders with a population-based cohort of 1023 adults with intellectual disabilities. Psychological Medicine. 2007;**37**(6):873-882

[43] Treppner P. Genetics and mental retardation syndromes. A new look at behaviour and interventions. Journal of Applied Research in Intellectual Disabilities. 2001;**14**(4):418-420

[44] Aylward EH, Li Q, Honeycutt NA, Warren AC, Pulsifer MB, Barta PE, et al. MRI volumes of the hippocampus and amygdala in adults with Down's syndrome with and without dementia. American Journal of Psychiatry. 1999;**156**(4):564-568

[45] Pinter JD, Eliez S, Schmitt JE, Capone GT, Reiss AL. Neuroanatomy of Down's syndrome: A high-resolution MRI study. American Journal of Psychiatry. 2001;**158**(10):1659-1665

[46] Seidl R, Kaehler S, Prast H, Singewald N, Cairns N, Gratzer M, et al. Serotonin (5-HT) in brains of adult patients with Down syndrome. J. Neural Transm. 1999; **57**(suppl.):221-232

[47] Myers BA, Pueschel SM. Major depression in a small group of adults with down syndrome. Research in Developmental Disabilities. 1995;**16**(4):285-299

[48] Jap SN, Ghaziuddin N. Catatonia among adolescents with down syndrome: A review and 2 case reports. The Journal of ECT. 2011;**27**(4):334-337

[49] Cooper S-A, Collacott RA. Clinical features and diagnostic criteria of depression in Down's syndrome. The British Journal of Psychiatry. 1994;**165**(3):399-403

[50] Janzing J, Teunisse R, Bouwens P, van't Hof M, Zitman F. Mood and motivation disturbance in elderly subjects with and without dementia: A replication study. The Journal of Nervous and Mental Disease. 1999;**187**(2):117-119

[51] Shott SR, Amin R, Chini B, Heubi C, Hotze S, Akers R. Obstructive sleep apnea: Should all children with down syndrome be tested? Archives of Otolaryngology–Head & Neck Surgery. 2006;**132**(4):432-436

[52] Byrne C, Seyfort B. Complications in the diagnosis and treatment of depression in persons with Down syndrome. The NADD Bulletin. 1998;**1**:103-106

[53] Torr J, D'Abrera JC. Maintenance electroconvulsive therapy for depression with catatonia in a young woman with down syndrome. The Journal of ECT. 2014;**30**(4):332-336

[54] Lindsay WR, Howells L, Pitcaithly D. Cognitive therapy for depression with individuals with intellectual disabilities. Psychology and Psychotherapy: Theory, Research and Practice. 1993;**66**(2):135-141

[55] Gensheimer PM, Meighen KG, McDougle CJECT. In an adolescent with down syndrome and treatment-refractory major depressive disorder. Journal of Developmental and Physical Disabilities. 2002;**14**(3):291-295

[56] LaiMC L, Baron-Cohen S. Autism. 2014;**383**(9920):896-910

[57] Dressler A, Perelli V, Bozza M, Bargagna S. The autistic phenotype in down syndrome: Differences in adaptive behaviour versus down syndrome alone and autistic disorder alone. Functional Neurology. 2011;**26**(3):151

[58] Rasmussen P, Börjesson O, Wentz E, Gillberg C. Autistic disorders in down syndrome: Background factors and clinical correlates. Developmental Medicine and Child Neurology. 2001;**43**(11):750-754

[59] Carter JC, Capone GT, Kaufmann WE. Neuroanatomic correlates of autism and stereotypy in children with down syndrome. Neuroreport. 2008;**19**(6):653-656

[60] Ghaziuddin M, Tsai LY, Ghaziuddin N. Autism in Down's syndrome: Presentation and diagnosis. Journal of Intellectual Disability Research. 1992;**36**(5):449-456

[61] Rachubinski AL, Hepburn S, Elias ER, Gardiner K, Shaikh TH. The co-occurrence of down syndrome and autism spectrum disorder: Is it because of additional genetic variations? Prenatal Diagnosis. 2017;**37**(1):31-36

[62] Mukaddes N. Eğitsel Tedavi Yaklaşımları-Bölüm8, In: Otizm spektrum bozuklukları tanı ve takip. Nobel Tıp Kitabevleri İstanbul. 2013:121-139

[63] Smith T. Applied behavior analysis and early intensive intervention. In: D. G. Amaral, G. Dawson, & D. H. Geschwind (Eds.), Autism spectrum disorders, New York, NY: Oxford University Press , 2011 (pp. 1037-1055)

[64] Towbin K, Riddle M. Obsessive-compulsive disorder. In: Child and Adolescent Psychiatry. Philadelphia: Lippincott Williams & Wilkins; 2002. p. 834-847

[65] Fineberg NA, Hengartner MP, Bergbaum CE, Gale TM, Gamma A, Ajdacic-Gross V, et al. A prospective population-based cohort study of the prevalence, incidence and impact of obsessive-compulsive symptomatology. International Journal of Psychiatry in Clinical Practice. 2013;**17**(3):170-178

[66] Abudy A, Juven-Wetzler A, Zohar J. Pharmacological management of treatment-resistant obsessive-compulsive disorder. CNS Drugs. 2011;**25**(7):585-596

[67] Pekrul SR, Fitzgerald KD. Memantine augmentation in a Down's syndrome adolescent with treatment-resistant obsessive-compulsive disorder. Journal of Child and Adolescent Psychopharmacology. 2015;**25**(7):593-595

[68] Thapar A, Pine DS, Leckman JF, Scott S, Snowling MJ, Taylor EA. Rutter's Child and Adolescent Psychiatry. John Wiley & Sons; West Susex. 2015

[69] Green SA, Berkovits LD, Baker BL. Symptoms and development of anxiety in children with or without intellectual disability. Journal of Clinical Child & Adolescent Psychology. 2015;**44**(1):137-144

[70] Kostyrko A, Hauser J, Rybakowski JK, Trzeciak WH. Screening of chromosomal region 21q22. 3 for mutations in genes associated with neuronal Ca2+ signalling in bipolar affective disorder. Acta Biochimica Polonica. 2006;**53**(2):317-320

[71] Roche S, Cassidy F, Zhao C, Badger J, Claffey E, Mooney L, et al. Candidate gene analysis of 21q22: Support for S100B as a susceptibility gene for bipolar affective disorder with psychosis. American Journal of Medical Genetics Part B: Neuropsychiatric Genetics. 2007;**144(**(8):1094-1096

[72] Craddock N, Owen MI. There an inverse relationship between Down's syndrome and bipolar affective disorder? Literature review and genetic implications. Journal of Intellectual Disability Research. 1994;**38**(6):613-620

[73] Dhossche DM, Wachtel LE. Catatonia is hidden in plain sight among different pediatric disorders: A review article. Pediatric Neurology. 2010;**43**(5):307-315

[74] Ghaziuddin N, Dhossche D, Marcotte K. Retrospective chart review of catatonia in child and adolescent psychiatric patients. Acta Psychiatrica Scandinavica. 2012;**125**(1):33-38

[75] Ghaziuddin N, Nassiri A, Miles JH. Catatonia in down syndrome; a treatable cause of regression. Neuropsychiatric Disease and Treatment. 2015;**11**:941

[76] Pommepuy N, Januel D. La catatonie: résurgence d'un concept. Une revue de la littérature internationale. Encephale. 2002;**27**:481-492

Chapter 3

Functional Neurogenomics: A New Approach to Study Cognitive Disability in Down Syndrome Brain

Felipe García-Vallejo,
Alejandra Rocío Rodríguez Ortiz,
Camila Azcárate Gómez, Meliza Santiago Ospina,
Julio César Montoya Villegas,
Adalberto Sánchez Gómez and
José María Satizábal Soto

Additional information is available at the end of the chapter

http://dx.doi.org/10.5772/intechopen.71057

Abstract

Functional neurogenomics is the interface between neurosciences knowledge and Omics sciences data. It characterizes, identifies, and analyzes expression of genes involved in the function of several structures of brain and cognition. Its major goal is to understand the main pathways of brain function, plasticity, and the etiopathogenesis of brain diseases. We have done an integrate analysis of global brain gene expression linked to cognitive disability in Down syndrome. It is a new approach to better understand the control of complex brain networks of gene expression involved in this syndrome. The objective of the chapter is to present computationally simulate data of global expression of 108 genes associated with cognitive disability and neuroplasticity from DNA microarray experiments of postmortem brain from normal controls and patients with Down syndrome. Some genes that were studied are involved in metabolic process and also promote hippocampal plasticity; interventions reawaken the neural plasticity may permit improved cognition. One of the striking findings was that some of the causes of dysregulation appear to result in the brain being trapped in an immature state of synaptic development. Understanding the functional neurogenomics of Down syndrome brain, emerge a new scenario to partially overcome cognitive disability through new prospective genomic therapies.

Keywords: brain, functional neurogenomics, omics sciences, Down syndrome, neuroplasticity, cognitive disability, data mining, DNA microarrays, computational biology

1. Introduction

Never before in brain research, the development of modern brain imaging technologies and the application of new brain analyses by using the Omics sciences, have provided new knowledge to explore not only the biological essence of human intelligence as well as the relationship between brain function and cognition. As results of such studies, actually we have an unprecedented state to understand the relationship between brain and intelligence [1]. Brain function and its dysfunction throughout life are determined by the interaction of genetic factors with internal and external environmental events, signals, and stimuli [2]. Most of this process occur early in life and exert many effects that persist throughout adulthood. In this scenario, the hippocampus is one of the targets that plays a crucial role in learning, memory storage and retrieval, and in general cognitive function; the study and management of hippocampal neuronal networks, open the real possibility to induce adaption by increasing its function, as a base for a real hippocampal rehabilitation combined therapies [3–5].

This chapter presents the main results of our investigations in the Down syndrome global gene expression from an integrative approach of functional neurogenomics (FN) as the interface of neurosciences and omics sciences (OS). NF emerges as an integrative research approach which applies several methods of computational sciences and OS strategies, to get understanding of how their gene-product interacts in complex networks and regulates the brain homeostasis. The information derived from the functional neurogenomics approach, could serve in the future, to develop new promising therapeutic protocols and genome editing strategies for trustworthy cognitive rehabilitation based on the hippocampal neuroplasticity [6–9].

2. Generalities of Down syndrome

Down syndrome (DS) is the most common aneuploidy in children caused by an extra 21 chromosome, affecting worldwide 1 in 600 live births and 1 in 150 conceptions [10]; however, remarkable differences are registered among countries that depend on sociocultural variables [11]. The triplication of genes on HSA21 causes a wide spectrum of neurological phenotypes in DS, including intellectual and cognitive disabilities. Patients with DS display not only delayed linguistic skills and a variable degrees of cognitive and intellectual disabilities, but also behavioral issues such as attention-deficit disorder (ADD, sometimes with hyperactivity) and autism spectrum disorder (ASD) [12–16]. The cognitive impairments extend further after development, as individuals with DS are more prone to develop Alzheimer's type dementia [17]. In addition, patients with DS are susceptible to epilepsy in the form of infantile spasms and tonic-clonic seizures with myoclonus at early ages [16].

It was reported that brain of Down syndrome has a reduction of size and diminishing number of neuron density. Part of the cognitive dysfunction in DS, lies not only in the progressive neuronal degeneration/cell death and impaired neurogenesis seen in this developmental and degenerative disorder, but also in the reduction in dendrite formation and spine density, which result in a disruption of synaptic function. These pathological abnormalities in humans are, in part, replicated in DS animal models which show defects in learning, social interactions, memory, and seizures [18–22].

http://dx.doi.org/10.5772/intechopen.71057

3. Functional neurogenomics: the systemic integration of brain global gene expression

The spectacular advances in OS, had led to obtain comprehensive global information regarding the transcriptome of some neurological diseases [23]. In this regard, the use of DNA microarrays to study global transcription is widely spread. This methodology has allowed performing comprehensive analysis of changes in transcriptional expression of many genes associated with the pathophysiology of DS [24]. In addition, previous studies have shown the importance of using postmortem brain tissue to analyze the transcriptome of different conditions and different regions of the human brain including those individuals with DS [25]. The gene expression profile of the central nervous system (CNS) is unique. At least 30–50% of approximately 22,000 known protein-coding genes are expressed across all structures of the human brain [26]. Moreover, the human brain has the highest level of gene expression compared with other mammal species [27]. Neurogenomics research applies genomic strategies to identify and analyze genes that are involved in the function of nervous system. One of the main goals is to build a really systemic approach that contributes to explain the brain development, function, plasticity, and associated diseases [6, 7, 28, 29].

As shown in **Figure 1**, the major goal in functional neurogenomics is to analyze the global gene expression among different structures of the brain in order to identify the normal regulation of transcription and characterize genes associated with several neurological pathologies with cognitive and intellectual disabilities phenotypes [28–31].

The functional neurogenomic analysis starts with planning of global gene expression in brain. In this sense, DNA microarray experiments are a powerful experimental tool to study the transcriptome profile of brain which varies within specific regions and changes with age and with internal and external environmental conditions [32, 33].

DNA microarray experiments generate large amounts of data; for example, in a gene expression microarray study, 22,000 genes x 100 samples will generate 2.2 million data points. This terabyte amount data of information is necessary to be analyzed by computational simulation procedures that use bioinformatics analysis tools to get information about the spatial and temporal gene expression. Moreover, the bioinformatics analysis permits to extract information about genes which are expressed in normal and pathological samples of postmortem brains [34, 35].

In addition, genomic experiments are often noisy and are not normally distributed, and usually contain missing values in the expression matrix. To overcome such problem and to obtain biological relevant interpretations of the genome expression data, robust biostatistical analyses are required [36, 37]. In general, statistical analyses of genomic data can be divided into two major categories: supervised and unsupervised methods [36]. Supervised analysis is used to identify genes that are differentially expressed between groups of samples, as well as to find genes that can be used to accurately predict the characteristics of groups. The unsupervised approaches characterize genomic data without prior input or knowledge of predetermined pattern. Unsupervised analysis is used to identify internal structure in the genomic data set. The most commonly used unsupervised analysis tool is Hierarchical clustering and Principal Components Analysis (PCA) [37].

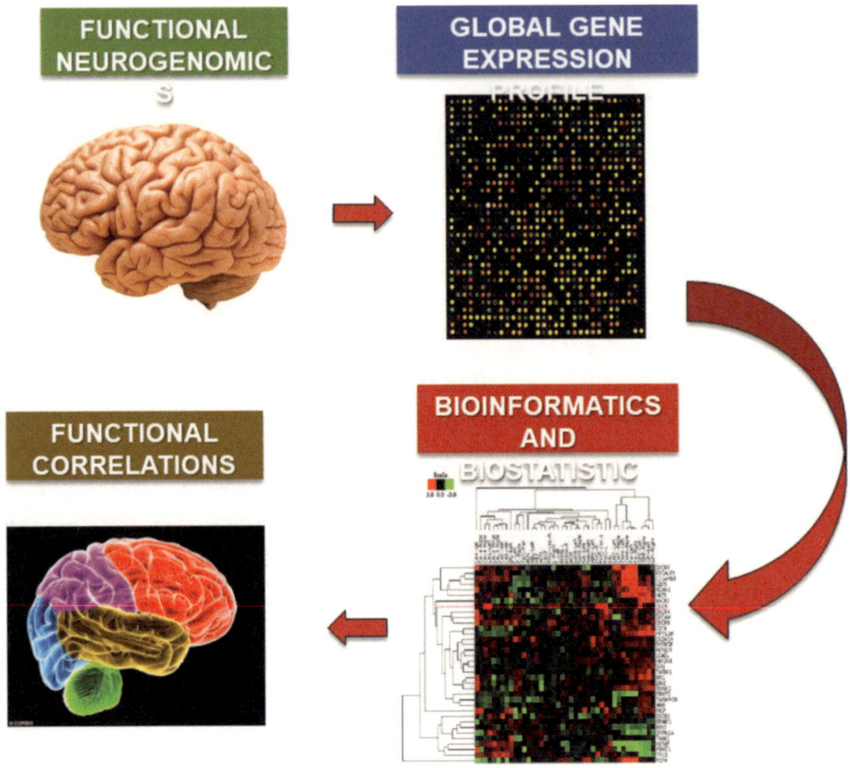

Figure 1. The experimental and analytical procedures applies in functional neurogenomics. The flow of procedures starts with the analysis of global gene expression profiles, using the technology of DNA microarray, which is followed by a trend of bioinformatics and statistical analysis of the results of the big data generated by DNA microarray experiments. As a result of the integrative analysis, the functional correlation between global gene expression and several interaction processes are obtained.

The final result of the flow of analytical process previously described, is to correlate the gene expression profiles variation within specific regions of the brain to obtain a better knowledge about the functional correlations. In this sense, DNA microarray experiments showed that the transcriptome profile of the CNS is specific of brain structure and also the signals that modulate it [38, 39].

4. Cognitive disability and neuroplasticity: our main approach

Cognition refers to the mental processes that are involved in acquiring knowledge and comprehension. These processes include thinking, knowing, remembering, judging, and problem solving. All of them are higher level functions of the brain and encompass language, imagination, perception, and planning [40]. Neuroplasticity is the ability of the nervous system to adapt to different environmental conditions and stimuli; it requires a well-conserved and flexible repertoire of molecular mechanisms [41]. Neural plasticity, allows neurons to regenerate both anatomically as well as functionally, in a process call neurogenesis; also to form new synaptic connections—synaptogenesis, and in some cases of new dendrites generation—dendritogenesis [42, 43]. Because neuroplasticity is based on the ability of brain to recover and restructure itself, it allows us to consider that its adaptive potential to recover after disorders or injuries, would be a point of departure for developing therapeutic strategies toward reducing the effects of altered structures due to cognitive associated pathologies including DS among others [44].

The point of departure of our studies lies in the fact that a failure in the crosstalk between cognitive process and neuroplasticity would be a major effector for cognitive disability (CD) in DS brain [45–48]. Some genetic mechanisms or even alteration of brain development homeostasis has important neurodevelopmental consequences produced by CD [49].

4.1. Our methodological approach

In order to test our proposal, the initial approach started with a bibliographic search of full papers in PubMed of publications reported neuroplasticity and CD in Down syndrome. We used the following crossed descriptors to perform that search: DS, neuroplasticity and cognition and cognitive disability, and genes associated. We filtered six full papers describing genes that involved in cognition and neuroplasticity in DS. Information consigned in this article led us to pick up 106 genes involved in neuroplasticity and cognitive process such as memory and learning. Those genes were the initial background to perform our computational simulations and identify their functional roles in several structures of brain cortex. Moreover from gender and age gene expression values, we obtain data about their temporal and spatial regulations. The list and main characteristics of selected genes are consigned in Supplementary **Table 1**.

As a source to calculate the values of expression for selected gene, this initial bibliographic search was crossed with DNA microarray experiments consigned in the database of GEO DataSet of NCBI (https://www.ncbi.nlm.nih.gov/gds/). Combining the descriptors: Down syndrome and global transcription and neuroplasticity and cognition and brain, we found nine DNA microarray experiments. However, only one of them fitted the statistical significance sample size to obtain trustable information about the functional neurogenomics in DS.

We used the log10 transformed expression values of a DNA microarray experiment whose registration code and free access in the GEO database was GSE59630 (http://www.ncbi.nlm.nih.gov/geo/query/acc.cgi?acc=GSE59630), previously deposited by Olmos et al. [50]. The microarray experiment selected included gene expression data of 47,000 probes from 58 DS patients (25 females and 33 males) and 58 healthy controls (25 females and 33 males) of post-mortem brain samples classified by gender and age, and in 11 structures of cerebral cortex.

4.2. Functional analysis

Free use Cytoscape 3.2 open software platform was used for visualizing and analyzing the genetic interaction networks among the selected human genes associated with cognition and neuroplasticity processes. Biological Networks Gene Ontology v2.6 plugin (BiNGO

ID	Gen symbol	Name	Locus	Function—gene ontology (GO)
90	ACVR1	Activin A receptor type 1	2q24.1	ATP binding
9509	ADAMTS2	ADAM metallopeptidase with thrombospondin type 1 motif 2	5q35.3	Metalloendopeptidase activity, metallopeptidase activity
9370	ADIPOQ	Adiponectin	3q27.3	Cytokine activity, hormone activity
152	ADRA2C	Adrenoceptor alpha 2C	4p16.3	Alpha-2A adrenergic receptor binding, epinephrine binding
8906	AP1G2	Adaptor related protein complex 1 gamma 2 subunit	14q11.2	Protein transporter activity
361	AQP4	Aquaporin 4	18q11.2	Protein binding
10317	B3GALT5	Beta-1,3-galactosyltransferase 5	21q22.2	Protein glycosylation
25825	BACE2	Beta-site APP-cleaving enzyme 2	21q22.2–q22.3	Amyloid-beta metabolic process
627	BDNF	Brain-derived neurotrophic factor	11p14.1	Neurotrophin TRKB receptor binding
666	BOK	BCL2 family apoptosis regulator	2q37.3	BH domain binding
54014	BRWD1	Bromodomain and WD repeat domain containing 1	21q22.2	Cytoskeleton organization
55969	C20orf24	Chromosome 20 open reading frame 24	20q11.23	Olfactory receptor activity
114041	B3GALT5-AS1	B3GALT5 antisense RNA 1	21q22.2	Putative uncharacterized
721	C4B	Complement C4B	6p21.33	Carbohydrate binding, endopeptidase inhibitor activity
23562	CLDN14	Claudin 14	21q22.13	Protein complex assembly
54102	CLIC6	Chloride intracellular channel 6	21q22.12	NOT glutathione metabolic process
1277	COL1A1	Collagen type I alpha 1 chain	17q21.33	Protease binding, extracellular matrix structural constituent, protein binding
1278	COL1A2	Collagen type I alpha 2 chain	7q21.3	SMAD binding, identical protein binding
1476	CSTB	Cystatin B	21q22.3	Adult locomotory behavior
7852	CXCR4	C-X-C motif chemokine receptor 4	2q22.1	C-C chemokine binding
51523	CXXC5	CXXC finger protein 5	5q31.2	Sequence-specific DNA binding, signal transducer activity, transcription factor binding
147991	DPY19L3	DPY-19-like 3	19q13.11	Mannosyltransferase activity, transferase activity
1812	DRD1	Dopamine receptor D1	5q35.2	Dopamine binding

ID	Gen symbol	Name	Locus	Function—gene ontology (GO)
3920	DSCAM	DS cell adhesion molecule	21q22.2	Nervous system development, Locomotory behavior, dendrite morphogenesis
10311	DSCR3	DSCR3 arrestin fold containing	21q22.13	Intracellular protein transport
53820	DSCR6	Ripply transcriptional repressor 3	21q22.13	Negative regulation of cell proliferation
84677	DSCR8	Down syndrome critical region 8 (non-protein coding)	21q22.13	Biological_process
1846	DUSP4	Dual specificity phosphatase 4	8p12	MAP kinase serine/threonine phosphatase activity
1859	DYRK1A	Dual specificity tyrosine phosphorylation regulated kinase 1A	21q22.13	Circadian rhythm
1958	EGR1	Early growth response 1	5q31.2	RNA polymerase II regulatory region sequence-specific DNA binding
2078	ERG	ERG, ETS transcription factor	21q22.2	Cell proliferation
2114	ETS2	ETS proto-oncogene 2, transcription factor	21q22.2	Skeletal system development
2199	FBLN2	Fibulin 2	3p25.1	Extracellular matrix binding, calcium ion binding
252995	FNDC5	Fibronectin type III domain containing 5	1p35.1	Hormone activity, molecular_function
2487	FRZB	Frizzled-related protein	2q32.1	Wnt-activated receptor activity, G protein-coupled receptor activity
2670	GFAP	Glial fibrillary acidic protein	17q21.31	Structural constituent of cytoskeleton, protein binding
2719	GPC3	Glypican 3	Xq26.2	Heparan sulfate proteoglycan binding, peptidyl-dipeptidase inhibitor activity
10457	GPNMB	Glycoprotein nmb	7p15.3	Integrin binding, heparin binding, chemoattractant activity
3141	HLCS	Holocarboxylase synthetase	21q22.13	Enzyme binding
3150	HMGN1	High mobility group nucleosomal binding domain 1	21q22.2	Transcription-coupled nucleotide-excision repair
9456	HOMER1	Homer scaffolding protein 1	5q14.1	G protein-coupled glutamate receptor binding
9454	HOMER3	Homer scaffolding protein 3	19p13.11	G protein-coupled glutamate receptor binding
3479	IGF1	Insulin-like growth factor 1	12q23.2	Growth factor activity, hormone activity, insulin-like growth factor receptor binding, insulin-like growth factor receptor binding

ID	Gen symbol	Name	Locus	Function—gene ontology (GO)
3488	IGFBP5	Insulin-like growth factor binding protein 5	2q35	Fibronectin binding, protein binding
3489	IGFBP6	Insulin-like growth factor binding protein 6	12q13.13	Growth factor binding, receptor binding
3600	IL15	Interleukin 15	4q31.21	Cytokine activity, cytokine receptor binding
3623	INHA	Inhibin alpha subunit	2q35	Cytokine activity, growth factor activity
3708	ITPR1	Inositol 1,4,5-trisphosphate receptor 1	3p26.1	Calcium channel inhibitor activity
170850	KCNG3	Potassium voltage-gated channel modifier subfamily G member 3	2p21	Delayed rectifier potassium channel activity
3772	KCNJ15	Potassium voltage-gated channel subfamily J member 15	21q22.13-q22.2	Potassium ion import
3775	KCNK1	Potassium two pore domain channel subfamily K member 1	1q42.2	Inward rectifier potassium channel activity
57576	KIF17	Kinesin family member 17	1p36.12	Microtubule motor activity, ATP binding, microtubule binding,
7071	KLF10	Kruppel-like factor 10	8q22.3	RNA polymerase II core promoter proximal region sequence-specific DNA binding
11202	KLK8	Kallikrein related-peptidase 8	19q13.41	Serine-type endopeptidase activity
150082	LCA5L	LCA5L, lebercilin like	21q22.2	Protein binding
9663	LPIN2	Lipin 2	18p11.31	Phosphatidate phosphatase activity
4058	LTK	Leukocyte receptor tyrosine kinase	15q15.1	ATP binding, protein binding
4147	MATN2	Matrilin 2	8q22.1-q22.2	Calcium ion binding
4239	MFAP4	Microfibril associated protein 4	17p11.2	Protein binding
283078	MKX	Mohawk homeobox	10p12.1	Sequence-specific DNA binding
25902	MTHFD1L	Methylenetetrahydrofolate dehydrogenase (NADP+ dependent) 1 like	6q25.1	Formate-tetrahydrofolate ligase activity, methylenetetrahydrofolate dehydrogenase (NADP+) activity
1463	NCAN	Neurocan	19p13.11	Calcium ion binding
4885	NPTX2	Neuronal pentraxin 2	7q22.1	Carbohydrate binding
51299	NRN1	Neuritin 1	6p25.1	C-terminal protein lipidation
51559	NT5DC3	5′-Nucleotidase domain containing 3	12q23.3	Metal ion binding
4908	NTF3	Neurotrophin 3	12p13.31	Chemoattractant activity, neurotrophin p75 receptor binding

http://dx.doi.org/10.5772/intechopen.71057

ID	Gen symbol	Name	Locus	Function—gene ontology (GO)
64881	PCDH20	Protocadherin 20	13q21.2	RNA binding, calcium ion binding
5121	PCP4	Purkinje cell protein 4	21q22.2	Positive regulation of neuron differentiation
5179	PENK	Proenkephalin	8q12.1	Neuropeptide hormone activity
51227	PIGP	Phosphatidylinositol glycan anchor biosynthesis class P	21q22.13	Preassembly of GPI anchor in ER membrane
130271	PLEKHH2	Pleckstrin homology, MyTH4 and FERM domain containing H2	2p21	Actin binding, identical protein binding
57460	PPM1H	Protein phosphatase, Mg2+/Mn2+ dependent 1H	12q14.1-q14.2	Phosphoprotein phosphatase activity, protein serine/threonine phosphatase activity
3275	PRMT2	Protein arginine methyltransferase 2	21q22.3	Developmental cell growth
8624	PSMG1	Proteasome assembly chaperone 1	21q22.2	Proteasome assembly
754	PTTG1IP	PTTG1 interacting protein	21q22.3	Protein import into nucleus
51655	RASD1	RAS related dexamethasone induced 1	17p11.2	GTPase activity, GTP binding
10633	RASL10A	RAS like family 10 member A	22q12.2	Signal transduction, small GTPase mediated signal transduction
1827	RCAN1	Regulator of calcineurin 1	21q22.12	Central nervous system development
5997	RGS2	Regulator of G protein signaling 2	1q31.2	G-protein alpha-subunit binding
85397	RGS8	Regulator of G protein signaling 8	1q25.3	GTPase activator activity
56475	RPRM	Reprimo, TP53 dependent G2 arrest mediator homolog	2q23.3	Protein binding
861	RUNX1	Runt related transcription factor 1	21q22.12	Peripheral nervous system neuron development
347735	SERINC2	Serine incorporator 2	1p35.2	L-serine transmembrane transporter activity
5271	SERPINB8	Serpin family B member 8	18q22.1	Serine-type endopeptidase inhibitor activity
6450	SH3BGR	SH3 domain binding glutamate rich protein	21q22.2	Positive regulation of signal transduction
6470	SHMT1	Serine hydroxymethyltransferase 1	17p11.2	L-allo-threonine aldolase activity, glycine hydroxymethyltransferase activity
6493	SIM2	Single-minded family bHLH transcription factor 2	21q22.13	Embryonic pattern specification
6574	SLC20A1	Solute carrier family 20 member 1	2q14.1	High-affinity inorganic phosphate:sodium symporter activity
65012	SLC26A10	Solute carrier family 26 member 10	12q13.3	Anion:anion antiporter activity

ID	Gen symbol	Name	Locus	Function—gene ontology (GO)
57709	SLC7A14	Solute carrier family 7 member 14	3q26.2	Amino acid transmembrane transporter activity
114826	SMYD4	SET and MYND domain containing 4	17p13.3	Metal ion binding, methyltransferase activity
6651	SON	SON DNA binding protein	21q22.11	Negative regulation of apoptotic process
6664	SOX11	SRY-box 11	2p25.2	RNA polymerase II core promoter sequence-specific DNA binding
8869	ST3GAL5	ST3 beta-galactoside alpha-2,3-sialyltransferase 5	2p11.2	Beta-galactoside (CMP) alpha-2,3-sialyltransferase activity
27090	ST6GALNAC4	ST6 N-acetylgalactosaminide alpha-2,6-sialyltransferase 4	9q34.11	Alpha-N-acetylgalactosaminide alpha-2,6-sialyltransferase activity
7058	THBS2	Thrombospondin 2	6q27	Heparin binding, protein binding
7059	THBS3	Thrombospondin 3	1q22	Heparin binding, calcium ion binding
7074	TIAM1	T-cell lymphoma invasion and metastasis 1	21q22.11	Neuron projection extension
757	TMEM50B	Transmembrane protein 50B	21q22.11	Biological_process
7109	TRAPPC10	Trafficking protein particle complex 10	21q22.3	Early endosome to Golgi transport
10098	TSPAN5	Tetraspanin 5	4q23	Enzyme binding
7267	TTC3	Tetratricopeptide repeat domain 3	21q22.13	Protein K48-linked ubiquitination
84959	UBASH3B	Ubiquitin associated and SH3 domain containing B	11q24.1	Identical protein binding, phosphoprotein binding
221044	UCMA	Upper zone of growth plate and cartilage matrix associated	10p13	Negative regulation of osteoblast differentiation
7422	VEGFA	Vascular endothelial growth factor A	6p21.1	Chemoattractant activity, cytokine activity
7485	WRB	Tryptophan rich basic protein	21q22.2	Tail-anchored membrane protein insertion into ER membrane

Table 1. Description of genes associated with neuroplasticity and cognition. Information taken from the NCBI—Genbank platform (Supplementary table).

tool) was used to search which gene ontology (GO) categories are significantly overrepresented in a set of genes. A hypergeometric test was applied to determine which categories were significantly represented (P-value < 0.05); significant values were adjusted for multiple hypotheses testing using the Bonferroni family wise error rate correction [51]. From network analyzer plugin of the Max Planck Institute Informatik, network topology parameters were calculated.

4.3. Z-score transformation

The raw intensity data for each gene in the DNA microarray experiment was log10 transformed and then used for the calculation of Z score [52]. Z scores were calculated by subtracting the mean log gene intensities (within a single experiment) from the log intensity data for each gene, and dividing that result by the SD of all measured log intensities, according to the Z-score transformation (1):

$$Z - score = \frac{(Log\ intensity\ of\ G - mean\ log intensity\ G \ldots Gn)}{Standard\ deviation\ log G \ldots Gn} \tag{1}$$

All Z-score values were normalized on a linear scale $-3.0 < 0 > +3.0$. In this, the corresponding gene is overexpressed if the value of Z-score is greater than zero; on the contrary, it is underexpressed, if its value is negative.

4.4. Multivariate statistical analysis

Nonparametric analyses for comparing median values of Z-score were performed among gender and age variables between DS patients and healthy control. Wilcoxon signed-rank test was used to calculate differences between medians of two samples.

Data of Z-score values of samples from DS and controls were compared to establish significant difference in gender in DS and controls and by age ranks since 16 weeks of gestation to 6 months; since 7 months up to 1 year; 2–3 years; 10–19 years; and 22 years and older groups. Moreover, Z-scores for the genes included in the study, were compared between DS and control samples in 11 structures of brain cortex including: dorsolateral prefrontal cortex (DFC), visual cortex (V1C), cerebellar cortex (CBC), orbitofrontal cortex (OFC), ventral frontal cortex (VFC), inferior temporal cortex (ITC), hippocampus (HIP), medial frontal cortex (MFC), somatosensory cortex (S1C), inferior parietal cortex (IPC), and superior temporal cortex (STC). To perform the HCA, Euclidean distance was used as a measure of distance between DS and control samples of Z-score values in several structures of brain cortex; $p < 0.05$ was defined as a threshold [53].

5. Our results

5.1. Protein network and gene interactions

A total of 3135 protein interactions among genes associated with cognition and neuroplasticity process expressed in brains of DS subjects were recorded (**Figure 2A** and **B**). The central proteins of the main node of the network corresponded to RUNX1 (runt related transcription factor 1) at 21q22.12; SON (SON DNA binding protein) at 21q22.11; RGS2 (regulator of G protein signaling 2) at 1q31.2; UBASH3B (ubiquitin associated and SH3 domain containing B) at 11q24.1; DYRK1A (dual specificity tyrosine phosphorylation regulated kinase 1A) at 21q22.13; GFAP (glial fibrillary acidic protein) at 17q21.31; TIAM1 (T-cell lymphoma

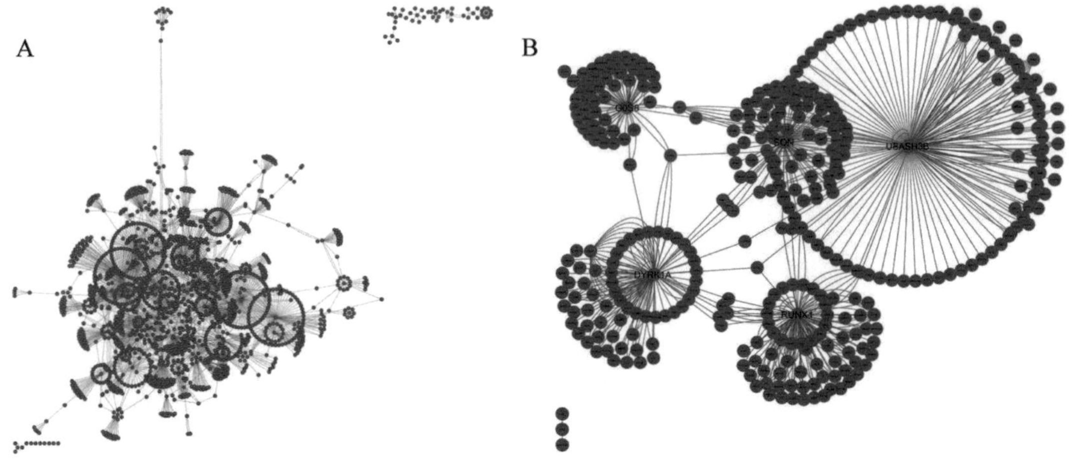

Figure 2. Protein-protein interaction (PPI) networks of genes associated with cognition and neuroplasticity constructed from data experiments of DNA microarray of genes expressed in Down syndrome postmortem brain samples. Data of log2 intensity values were obtained from DNA microarray experiment by Olmos-Serrano et al. [50], (GEO Dataset accession GSE59630). (A) Full network of 108 genes associated with cognition and neuroplasticity; (B) sub-network showing five of the major nodes found in the original network; Cytoscape 3.2 program was used to generate the graphical representation of built networks; UBASH3B, ubiquitin associated and SH3 domain containing B; SON, SON DNA binding protein; G0S8 (RGS2), regulator of G protein signaling 2; DYRK1A, dual specificity tyrosine phosphorylation regulated kinase 1A; RUNX1, runt-related transcription factor 1.

invasion and metastasis 1) at 21q22.11; and THBS3 (thrombospondin-3) at 1q22. The most important topological parameters of the network were: clustering coefficient with a value of 0.33; average number of neighbors 2367; network density 0.001 and 12 connected components (**Table 2**).

From GeneMANIA Cytoscape plugin, we identified the top five functions of that genes. They corresponded to regulation of behavior, behavior, muscle cell migration, hormone activity, and G coupled glutamate receptor.

5.2. Differential gene expression in post-mortem brains of DS patients

Overall no statistical differences between the median values in Z-score of the 108 gene in controls and DS patients were recorded (Controls 0.2869 vs. DS 0.3318; Wilcoxon rank test $p > 0.05$). However, significant differences in the medians of Z-score in some genes were determined. Thus, in the DS brains, the overexpression levels corresponded to genes CXXC5 (Controls −1.2376 vs. DS 0.7492), EGR1 (controls −1.2266 vs. DS 0.5442), and NCAN (controls −1.2901 vs. DS 0.5440).

The main GO categories of brains processes associated with DS involved in its etiopathogenesis included: respiratory electron transport chain (3.31E − 41), positive regulation of cell death (1.17E − 39), positive regulation of release of cytochrome c from mitochondria (9.19E − 37), negative regulation of cell motility involved in cerebral cortex radial glia guided migration

Topological parameter	Value
Clustering coefficient	0.33
Connected components	12
Network diameter	12
Network radius	1
Network centralization	0.056
Shortest paths	3.454.424 (93%)
Characteristics path length	5.340
Avg. number of neighbors	2.367
Number of nodes	1919
Network density	0.001
Network heterogeneity	3.105
Isolated nodes	0
Number of self-loops	25
Multi-edge node pairs	595

Table 2. Values of the main topological parameters of the protein interaction network including 106 genes associated with cognitive and neuroplasticity process in brain of DS patients.

(5.20E − 35), telomere maintenance (1.16E − 34), negative regulation of angiogenesis (4.11E − 32), and axonogenesis (1.40E − 31) (**Table 3**). Moreover, focal adhesion (P-value 7.69E − 23) and neurotrophin signaling pathway (P-value 3.62E − 19) were also important pathways associated with cognitive and neuroplasticity process in brains of DS individuals.

5.3. Evaluation of gene expression by sex and age variables

We observed differential brain expression in 72 genes associated with CD among women and men. Medians of brain gene expression in men patients with DS were higher than in DS women ($p < 0.005$ Kruskal-Wallis test) (**Figure 4A**). Such difference were statically significant for the expression of DMXL2 (Z-score of men 1.33 vs. −1.75 in women); CAMTA1 (Z-score of men 1.16 vs. −1.73 in women); HCN1 (Z-score of 1.05 vs. −1.73 in women); and ATL1 (Z-score of men 0.85 vs. −1.73 in women). On the contrary, we recorded non-significant differences by gender in medians values of genes associated with neuroplasticity in brains of DS.

Global gene expression among the different ranks of age in DS brains was variable and dependent of the type of gene. However, slight differences of expression in brain genes associated with neuroplasticity process of Down syndrome and its age dependency were recorded in samples of DS brains in comparison with that of normal controls in age ranks since 16 weeks of gestation to more than 22 years old. It is noteworthy that DYRK1A, NCAM AND TSPN5 genes were under-expressed in prenatal brains (**Figure 3A–G**).

GO_ID	Process	P-value*
9987	Respiratory electron transport chain	3.31E – 41
48522	Positive regulation of cell death	1.17E – 39
48518	Positive regulation of release of cytochrome c from mitochondria	9.19E – 37
48523	Negative regulation of cell motility involved in cerebral cortex radial glia guided migration	5.20E – 35
44260	Telomere maintenance	1.16E – 34
48519	Negative regulation of angiogénesis	4.11E – 32
16043	Axonogenesis	1.40E – 31
43170	Glycoprotein biosynthetic process	3.33E – 30
10604	Positive regulation of telomerase activity	1.82E – 29
9893	Positive regulation of protein processing in phagocytic vesicle	5.01E – 28

*P-values were calculated using the correction of Bonferroni.
Ontology v2.6 plugin (BiNGO tool) was used to search gene ontology (GO) categories.

Table 3. The top 10 GO categories of brains processes associated with DS involved in its etiopathogenesis.

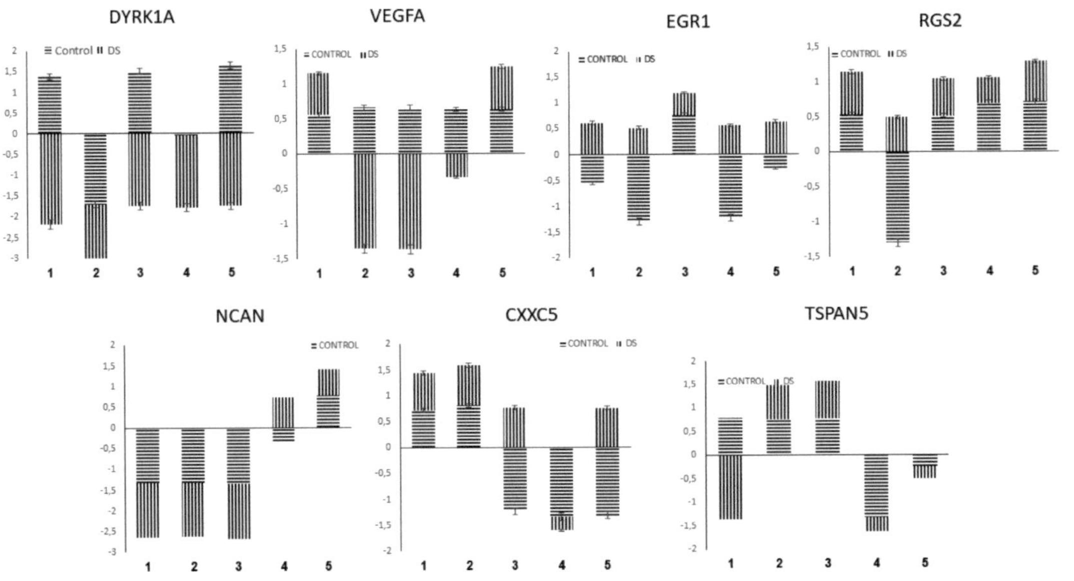

Figure 3. Differential values of median Z-score by age rank for six principal genes associated with cognitive disability and neuroplasticity expressed in brain samples of Down syndrome. (1) 16 Weeks of gestation to 6 months; (2) 7 months to 1 year; (3) 2–3 years; (4) 8–18 years; and (5) over 22 years of age. Y-axis values are the median of Z-score.

5.4. Gene expression in cerebral cortex

Some of the most differentially expressed genes across the cerebral cortex are shown in **Figure 4A–H**. In particular, expression in S1C showed significant differences for SERPIB8 (Control 0.2288 vs. DS −2.0288), SHMT1 (control 0.1542 vs. DS −2.1269) and THBSH3 (control

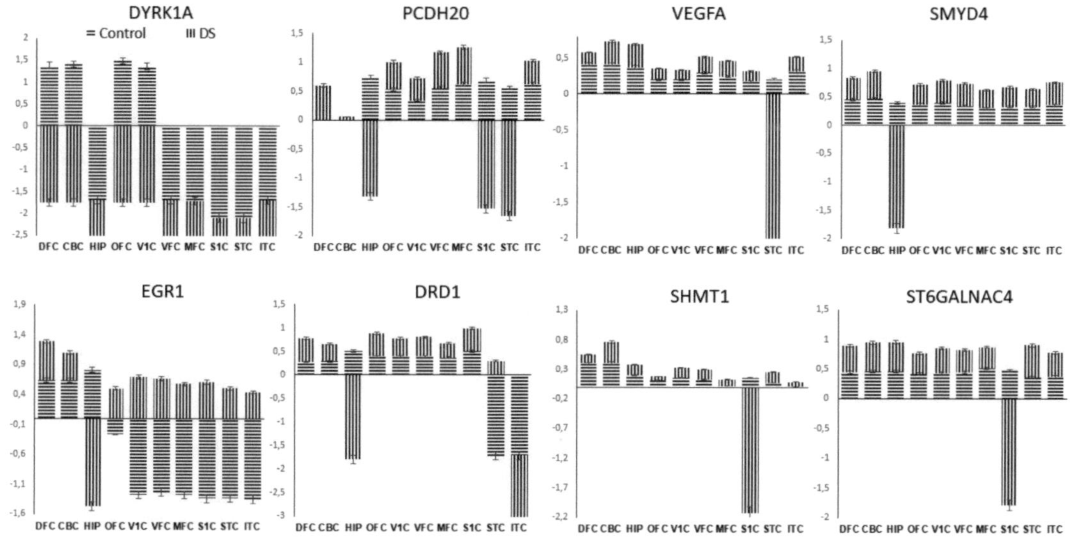

Figure 4. Differential gene expression in different structures of brain cortex of genes associated with cognitive disability and neuroplasticity in DS samples of brain. DFC, dorso lateral prefrontal cortex; V1C, visual cortex; CBC, cerebellar cortex; OFC, orbito frontal cortex; VFC, ventral frontal cortex; ITC, inferior temporal cortex; HIP, hippocampus; MFC, medial frontal; S1C, cortex somatosensory cortex; IPC, inferior parietal cortex and STC, superior temporal cortex. Y-axis values are the median of Z-score.

0.1542 vs. −2.0709) genes. In hippocampus, we recorded differential expression for EGR1 (control 0.8084 vs. DS −1.4648), SMYD4 (control 0.3946 vs. −1.8171), PCDH20 (control 0.7462 vs. DS −1.3194), DYRK1A (control 1.4284 vs. DS −1.7390), and VEGFA (control 0.6648 vs. DS −1.3280). In S1C, the most under expressed genes in Down syndrome were MFAP4 (control 0.1711 vs. DS −2.1461), BDNF (control 0.2136 vs. DS −2.1039), RGS8 (control 0.4013 vs. DS −1.9024), and SERINC2 (control 0.2584 vs. DS −1.8843). Finally in V1C, ADIPOQ (control −0.0035 vs. DS −2.1880), and TSPAN5 (control 0.7392 vs. DS −1.3315) were the most under-expressed genes in DS samples.

6. Discussion

In general, our results provided strong evidence to propose that in brains of DS, a fail in the cross talk of global expression between genes associated with cognition and neuroplasticity process (most of them located out of chromosome 21), is complex and is associated not only with pathological profiles but with gender, age, and is also dependent of the brain cortex structures. However, according with the functional roles, differential expression of particular groups of genes would cause a considerable impact on the metabolic pathways, in which they participate and are directly or indirectly involved in the regulation of molecular events associated with cognition and neuroplasticity in brain of patients with DS.

Overall, this study also support the hypothesis of a systemic imbalance of brain protein homeostasis, or proteostasis network as an important effect of trisomy not only in loci of chromosome 21 but also in genes located in other chromosomes [54]. Together our results and others collectively suggest that disturbance in the proteostasis network of cognitive and neuroplasticity process, could contribute to the accumulation of protein aggregates, such as amyloid deposits and NFTs, which occur very early in DS. It is likely that a sub-optimal functioning of degradative systems occur in DS neurons, which in turn provide the basis for further accumulation of toxic protein aggregates which have an indirect impact on the neuroplastic process in several structures of brain cortex [55, 56].

According to our results and with the information reviewed in literature, V-CAM1, SPTAN1, DYNC1H1, PAFAH1B1, H3F3A, ACVR1, THBS3, and TSPAN5 were the proteins with the highest number of protein interactions. All of them directly or even indirectly regulate several brain processes associated with cognition and neuroplasticity [57, 58]. In this sense, it is relevant to get more knowledge about the implication in those neurophysiological processes whose function is altered by either overexpression or by disruption in the network functional interaction architecture in DS brains.

For the first time, we obtain strong evidence that brain of male DS had, in general, a higher gene expression of cognitive and neuroplasticity process in comparison with that of females. The outstanding differences were specifically for DMXL2 (RKPM = 8.02 ± 1.61), CAMTA1 (RKPM = 4977 ± 1.246), HCN1 (RKPM = 4.88 ± 2.29), and ATL1 (RKPM = 34.764 ± 11.66) genes, all of them highly expressed in human brain. Previous evidence indicates that male-biased genes are highly enriched for genes involved in neurological and psychiatric disorders such as schizophrenia, bipolar disorder, Alzheimer's disease, and autism, while no such pattern was seen for the female-biased genes, suggesting that the differences in brain disorder susceptibility between males and females are likely rooted from the sex-biased gene expression regulation during brain development [59]. Moreover, it was previously reported that the excess of male cases with Down syndrome is not restricted to free trisomy 21 alone, but appears in translocation cases [60] and with the life expectancy found in males with DS, which is significantly greater in females [61]. Collectively, our and others analyses reveal the important role of sex-biased genes in brain development and neurodevelopmental disorders including the effects in cognitive disability in DS.

DYRK1A, BDNF, PENK, and DRD1 genes are strongly under-expressed in dorsolateral prefrontal cortex, hippocampus, orbitofrontal cortex, and ventral frontal cortex in subjects with DS in contrast with non-trisomic. Prefrontal cortex is implicated in planning complex cognitive behavior, personality expression, decision-making, and moderating social behavior [62], and also plays key roles in cell proliferation and survival, neuronal differentiation, synaptic plasticity, and neurodegeneration (for review, see [63, 64]). Supporting our proposal, it has been reported that DYRK1A/RCAN1 and NFAT lead to neurodevelopmental alterations that might have an impact not only in the brain size and neuronal density, but also in the altered common features found in patients with DS [65]. Additionally, a reduction of vesicular GABA transporter punctate specifically on parvalbumin-positive interneurons was identified [66, 67]. Overall, our results and others suggest that dysfunction of cortical fast-spiking interneurons might be central to the pathophysiology of DS.

The under-expression of key genes for brain function correlates with previous reports that showed that DS brains are smaller than normal brains and they exhibit neuronal deficits in several regions, including the cerebral cortex structures [68]. Moreover, infants with DS also present hypocellularity in this brain structure [69, 70], indicating that defects in prenatal development are a major determinant of the deficit in adults. Indeed, fewer cells and disorganized laminas are evident in the cerebral cortex of DS fetuses from as early as the second trimester of gestation [71, 72]. Altogether, the different lines of evidence support the hypothesis that DS brain is severely affected by the disturbance of proteostatic network, which is major responsible for the cerebral phenotype of DS.

Differential gene expression in hippocampus visual cortex, and somatosensory cortex of DYRK1A (dual specificity tyrosine-phosphorylation-regulated kinase 1A), TSPAN5 (tetraspanin 5), DRD1 (dopamine receptor D1), EGR1 (early growth response 1), GFAP (glial fibrillary acidic protein), and PENK (proenkephalin), which encode proteins that play important roles in several brain processes of cognition, learning and the maintenance of homeostasis, lead us to proposed them as functional potential predictors to follow up the homeostatic imbalance in DS brain.

Finally, this study showed that the integration of knowledge and use of cross talk between neurotranscriptomics and bioinformatics is a powerful work to develop transdisciplinary and systems biology studies to deal with many insight still remains to be solve in Down syndrome. We recommend continuing to study much deeper the complexity of interaction networks in the DS etiopathogenesis and brain homeostasis. On the other hand, our approach could serve as a starting point for the implementation of strategies to the management of cognitive and mental disabilities based on functional neurogenomics and the hippocampal neuroplasticity.

Author details

Felipe García-Vallejo[1]*, Alejandra Rocío Rodríguez Ortiz[2], Camila Azcárate Gómez[2], Meliza Santiago Ospina[2], Julio César Montoya Villegas[1], Adalberto Sánchez Gómez[1] and José María Satizábal Soto[1]

*Address all correspondence to: labiomol@gmail.com

1 Universidad del Valle, Cali, Colombia

2 Investigation group LABIOMOL- Universidad del Valle, Cali, Colombia

References

[1] Cairó O. Assessing relevance of external cognitive measures. Frontiers in Integrative Neuroscience. 2017;**11**:3. DOI: 10.3389/fnint.2017.00003

[2] McEwen BS. Stress and hippocampal plasticity. Annual Review of Neuroscience. 1999;**22**: 105-122. DOI: 10.1146/annurev.neuro.22.1.105

[3] Morris R. Developments of a water-maze procedure for studying spatial learning in the rat. Journal of Neuroscience Methods. 1984;**11**:47-60. DOI: 10.1016/0165-0270(84)90007-4

[4] Clark RE, Zola SM, Squire LR. Impaired recognition memory in rats after damage to the hippocampus. The Journal of Neuroscience. 2000;**20**:8853-8860

[5] Hollup SA, Kjelstrup KG, Hoff J, Moser MB, Moser EI. Impaired recognition of the goal location during spatial navigation in rats with hippocampal lesions. The Journal of Neuroscience. 2001;**21**:4505-4513

[6] Han G, Sun J, Wang J, Bai Z, Song F, Lei H. Genomics in neurological disorders. Genomics, Proteomics & Bioinformatics. 2014;**12**(4):156-163. DOI: 10.1016/j.gpb.2014.07.002

[7] Cardoso SD, Teles MC, Oliveira RF. Neurogenomic mechanisms of social plasticity. The Journal of Experimental Biology. 2015;**218**(Pt 1):140-149. DOI: 10.1242/jeb.106997

[8] Wendland JR, Ehlers MD. Translating neurogenomics into new medicines. Biological Psychiatry. 2016;**79**(8):650-656. DOI: 10.1016/j.biopsych.2015.04.027

[9] Heidenreich M, Zhang F. Applications of CRISPR-Cas systems in neuroscience. Nature Reviews Neuroscience. 2016;**17**(1):36-44. DOI: 10.1038/nrn.2015.2

[10] Hernandez D, Fisher EMC. Down syndrome genetics: Unravelling a multifactorial disorder. Human Molecular Genetics. 1996;**5**:1411-1416. DOI: 10.1093/hmg/5.Supplement_1.1411

[11] Stoll C, Alembik Y, Dott B, Roth MP. Study of DS in 238942 consecutive births. Annales de Génétique. 1998;**41**:44-51

[12] Capone G, Goyal P, Ares W, Lannigan E. Neurobehavioral disorders in children, adolescents, and young adults with Down syndrome. American Journal of Medical Genetics Part C: Seminars in Medical Genetics (Review). 2006;**142C**(3):158-172. DOI: 10.1002/ajmg.c.30097

[13] Coe DA, Matson JL, Russell DW, Slifer KJ, Capone GT, et al. Behavior problems of children with Down syndrome and life events. Journal of Autism and Developmental Disorders (Clinical Trial Controlled Clinical Trial). 1999;**29**(2):149-156. DOI: 10.1023/A:1023044711293

[14] Gath A, Gumley D. Behaviour problems in retarded children with special reference to Down's syndrome. The British Journal of Psychiatry: The Journal of Mental Science. 1986;**149**:156-161. DOI: 10.1192/bjp.149.2.156

[15] Kent L, Evans J, Paul M, Sharp M. Comorbidity of autistic spectrum disorders in children with Down syndrome. Developmental Medicine & Child Neurology (Case Reports). 1999;**41**(3):153-158. DOI: 10.1111/j.1469-8749.1999.tb00574.x

[16] Myers BA, Pueschel SM. Psychiatric disorders in persons with Down syndrome. The Journal of Nervous and Mental Disease. 1991;**179**(10):609-613. DOI: 10.1097/00005053-199110000-00004

[17] Lott IT. Down's syndrome, aging, and Alzheimer's disease: a clinical review. Annals of the New York Academy of Sciences (Research Support, U.S. Gov't, P.H.S. Review). 1982;**396**:15-27. DOI: 10.1111/j.1749-6632.1982.tb26840.x

[18] Cortez MA, Shen L, Wu Y, Aleem IS, Trepanier CH, et al. Infantile spasms and Down syndrome: A new animal model. Pediatric Research. 2009;**65**(5):499-503. DOI: 10.1203/PDR.0b013e31819d9076

[19] Coussons-Read ME, Crnic LS. Behavioral assessment of the Ts65Dn mouse, a model for Down syndrome: Altered behavior in the elevated plus maze and open field. Behavior Genetics. 1996;**26**(1):7-13. DOI: 10.1007/BF02361154

[20] Hyde LA, Frisone DF, Crnic LS. Ts65Dn mice, a model for Down syndrome, have deficits in context discrimination learning suggesting impaired hippocampal function. Behavioural Brain Research. 2001;**118**(1):53-60. DOI: 10.1016/S0166-4328(00)00313-2

[21] Reeves RH, Irving NG, Moran TH, Wohn A, Kitt C, et al. A mouse model for Down syndrome exhibits learning and behaviour deficits. Nature Genetics. 1995;**11**(2):177-184. DOI: 10.1038/ng1095-177

[22] Westmark CJ, Westmark PR, Malter JS. Alzheimer's disease and Down syndrome rodent models exhibit audiogenic seizures. Journal of Alzheimer's Disease (JAD). 2010;**20**(4):1009-1013. DOI: 10.3233/JAD-2010-100087

[23] Belichenko PV, Madani R, Rey-Bellet L, Pihlgren M, Becker A, Plassard A, et al. An anti-β-amyloid vaccine for treating cognitive deficits in a mouse model of Down syndrome. PLoS One. 2016;**11**(3):e0152471. DOI: 10.1371/journal.pone.0152471

[24] Kahlem P. Gene-dosage effect on chromosome 21 transcriptome in trisomy 21: Implication in Down syndrome cognitive disorders. Behavior Genetics. 2006 May;**36**(3):416-428. DOI: 10.1007/s10519-006-9053-z

[25] Ravid R. Biobanks for biomarkers in neurological disorders: The da Vinci bridge for optimal clinico-pathological connection. Journal of the Neurological Sciences. 2009;**283**(1-2):119-126. DOI: 10.1016/j.jns.2009.02.364

[26] Myers AJ, Gibbs JR, Webster JA, Rohrer K, Zhao A, Marlowe L, et al. A survey of genetic human cortical gene expression. Nature Genetics. 2007;**39**:1494-1499. DOI: 10.1038/ng.2007.16

[27] Enard W, Khaitovich P, Klose J, Zöllner S, Heissig F, Giavalisco P, et al. Intra- and interspecific variation in primate gene expression patterns. Science. 2002;**296**:340-343. DOI: 10.1126/science.1068996

[28] Boguski MS, Jones AR. Neurogenomics: At the intersection of neurobiology and genome sciences. Nature Neuroscience. 2004;**7**:429-433. DOI: 10.1038/nn1232

[29] Wendland JR, Ehlers MD. Translating Neurogenomics into new medicines. Biological Psychiatry. 2016 Apr 15;**79**(8):650-656. DOI: 10.1016/j.biopsych.2015.04.027

[30] Chow HM, Herrup K. Genomic integrity and the ageing brain. Nature Reviews. Neuroscience. 2015 Nov;**16**(11):672-684. DOI: 10.1038/nrn4020

[31] Montoya-Villegas JC, Soto-Girón J, Satizábal-Soto JM, Sánchez-Gómez A, García-Vallejo F. Genomic study of the critical region of chromosome 21 associated to Down syndrome. Colombia Médica. 2011;**42**:26-38

[32] Maze I, Shen L, Zhang B, et al. Nature neuroscience review: Analytical tools and current challenges in the modern era of Neuroepigenomics. Nature Neuroscience. 2014;**17**(11):1476-1490. DOI: 10.1038/nn.3816

[33] Dönertaş HM, İzgi H, Kamacıoğlu A, He Z, Khaitovich P, et al. Gene expression reversal toward pre-adult levels in the aging human brain and age-related loss of cellular identity. Scientific Reports 2017;**7**(1):5894. DOI: 10.1038/s41598-017-05927-4

[34] Santiago-Ospina M, Rodríguez A, Montoya JC, Sánchez A, Satizábal JM, García-Vallejo F. Gene expression of mental disability associated genes in brains of patients with Down syndrome. Revista de la Asociación Colombiana de *Ciencias* Biológicas (Col.). 2016;**28**:121-128

[35] Montoya JC, Fajardo D, Peña A, Sánchez A, Domínguez MC, Satizábal JM, García-Vallejo F. Global differential expression of genes located in the Down syndrome critical region in normal human brain. Colombia Médica. 2014;**45**(4):154-161

[36] Slonim DK. From patterns to pathways: Gene expression data analysis comes of age. Nature Genetics. 2002;**32**(Suppl):502-508. DOI: 10.1038/ng1033

[37] Allison DB et al. Microarray data analysis: From disarray to consolidation and consensus. Nature Reviews. Genetics. 2006;**7**(1):55-65. DOI: 10.1038/nrg1749

[38] Lodato MA, Woodworth MB, Lee S, Evrony GD, Mehta BK, et al. Somatic mutation in single human neurons tracks developmental and transcriptional history. Science. 2015;**350**(6256):94-98. DOI: 10.1126/science.aab1785

[39] Tsuji S. The neurogenomics view of neurological diseases. JAMA Neurology. 2013;**70**(6): 689-694. DOI: 10.1001/jamaneurol.2013.734

[40] Blomberg O. Concepts of cognition for cognitive engineering. The International Journal of Aviation Psychology. 2011;**21**:85-104. DOI: 10.1080/10508414.2011.537561

[41] Bennett EL, Diamond MC, Krech D, Rosenzweig MR. Chemical and anatomical plasticity of the brain. Science. 1964;**146**:610-619. DOI: 10.1126/science.146.3644.610

[42] Ming G, Song H. Adult neurogenesis in the mammalian brain: Significant answers and significant questions. Neuron. 2011;**70**(4):687-702. DOI: 10.1016/j.neuron.2011.05.001

[43] Vadodaria KC, Gage FH. SnapShot: Adult hippocampal neurogenesis. Cell. 2014;**156**(5): 1114-1114.e1. DOI: 10.1016/j.cell.2014.02.029

[44] Castilla-Ortega E, Pedraza C, Estivill-Torrús G, Santín LJ. When is adult hippocampal neurogenesis necessary for learning? Evidence from animal research. Reviews in the Neurosciences. 2011;**22**(3):267-283. DOI: 10.1515/rns.2011.027

[45] Winblad B, Palmer K, Kivipelto M. Mild cognitive impairment beyond controversies, towards a consensus: Report of the international working group on mild cognitive impairment. Journal of Internal Medicine. 2004;**256**:240-246. DOI: 10.1111/j.1365-2796.2004.01380.x

[46] American Psychiatric Association. Diagnostic and Statistical Manual of Mental Disorders (DSM-5). 5th ed. Washington, DC; 2013. DOI: 10.1176/appi.books.9780890425596

[47] Reiff HB, Gerber PJ, Ginsberg R. Definitions of learning disabilities from adults with learning disabilities: The Insiders' perspectives. Learning Disability Quarterly. 1993;**16**(2):114-125. DOI: 10.2307/1511133

[48] Maulik PK, Harbour CK. Epidemiology of intellectual disability. International Encyclopedia of Rehabilitation. Buffalo, Center for International Rehabilitation Research Information and Exchange; 2010. p. 1-12

[49] Chiurazzi P. Mental retardation: Is naming the real issue? American Journal of Medical Genetics. Part A. 2011;**155A**(5):974-975. DOI: 10.1002/ajmg.a.33950

[50] Olmos-Serrano JL, Kang HJ, Tyler WA, et al. Down syndrome developmental brain transcriptome reveals defective oligodendrocyte differentiation and myelination. Neuron. 2016;**89**(6):1208-1222. DOI: 10.1016/j.neuron.2016.01.042

[51] Maere S, Heymans K, Kuiper M. BiNGO: A cytoscape plug-in to assess overrepresentation of gene ontology categories in biological networks. Bioinformatics. 2005;**21**(16): 3448-3449. DOI: 10.1093/bioinformatics/bti551

[52] Cheadle C, Vawter MP, Freed WJ, Becker KG. Analysis of microarray data using Z score transformation. Journal of Molecular Diagnostics (JMD). 2003;**5**(2):73-81. DOI: 10.1016/S1525-1578(10)60455-2

[53] Cameron DA, Middleton FA, Chenn A, Olson EC. Hierarchical clustering of gene expression patterns in the Eomes+lineage of excitatory neurons during early neocortical development. BMC Neuroscience. 2012;**13**:90. DOI: 10.1186/1471-2202-13-90

[54] Labbadia J, Morimoto RI. The biology of proteostasis in aging and disease. Annual Review of Biochemistry. 2015;**84**:435-464. DOI: 10.1146/annurev-biochem-060614-033955

[55] Di Domenico F, Coccia R, Cocciolo A, Murphy MP, Cenini G, et al. Impairment of proteostasis network in Down syndrome prior to the development of Alzheimer's disease neuropathology: Redox proteomics analysis of human brain. Biochimica et Biophysica Acta. 2013;**1832**(8):1249-1259. DOI: 10.1016/j.bbadis.2013.04.013

[56] Aivazidis S, Coughlan CM, Rauniyar AK, Jiang H, Liggett LA, et al. The burden of trisomy 21 disrupts the proteostasis network in Down syndrome. PLoS One. Apr 21, 2017;**12**(4):e0176307. DOI: 10.1371/journal.pone.0176307

[57] Hole M, Winter MP, Wagner O, Exner M, Schillinger M, Arnold Z, et al. The impact of selectins on mortality in stable carotid atherosclerosis. Thrombosis and Haemostasis. 2015;**114**(3):632-638. DOI: 10.1160/TH14-12-1014

[58] Huang CW, Tsai MH, Chen NC, Chen WH, YT L, Lui CC, et al. Clinical significance of circulating vascular cell adhesion molecule-1 to white matter disintegrity in Alzheimer's dementia. Thrombosis and Haemostasis. 2015;**114**(6):1230-1234. DOI: 10.1160/TH14-11-0938

[59] Shi L, Zhang Z, Sex Biased SB. Gene expression profiling of human brains at major developmental stages. Scientific Reports. 2016;**6**:21181. DOI: 10.1038/srep21181

[60] Kovaleva NV. Sex ratio in Down syndrome. Tsitologiia i Genetika. 2002;**36**(6):54-69

[61] Glasson EJ, Sullivan SG, Hussain R, Petterson BA, Montgomery PD, Bittles AH. Comparative survival advantage of males with Down syndrome. American Journal of Human Biology. 2003;**15**(2):192-195. DOI: 10.1002/ajhb.10132

[62] Yang Y, Raine A. Prefrontal structural and functional brain imaging findings in antisocial, violent, and psychopathic individuals: A meta-analysis. Psychiatry Research. 2009;**174**(2):81-88. DOI: 10.1016/j.pscychresns.2009.03.012

[63] Pujol J, Del Hoyo L, Blanco-Hinojo L, De Sola S, Macià D, et al. Anomalous brain functional connectivity contributing to poor adaptive behavior in Down syndrome. Cortex. 2015;**64**:148-156. DOI: 10.1016/j.cortex.2014.10.012

[64] Dierssen M. Down syndrome: The brain in trisomic mode. Nature Reviews. Neuroscience. 2012;**13**:844-858. DOI: 10.1038/nrn3314

[65] Duchon A, Herault Y. DYRK1A, a dosage-sensitive gene involved in neurodevelopmental disorders, is a target for drug development in Down syndrome. Frontiers in Behavioral Neuroscience. 2016;**10**:104. DOI: 10.3389/fnbeh.2016.00104

[66] Ruiz-Mejias M, Martinez de Lagran M, Mattia M, Castano-Prat P, Perez-Mendez L, et al. Overexpression of Dyrk1A, a Down syndrome candidate, decreases excitability and impairs gamma oscillations in the prefrontal cortex. The Journal of Neuroscience. 2016;**36**(13):3648-3659. DOI: 10.1523/JNEUROSCI.2517-15.2016

[67] Thomazeau A, Lassalle O, Iafrati J, Souchet B, Guedj F, et al. Prefrontal deficits in a murine model overexpressing the Down syndrome candidate gene dyrk1a. The Journal of Neuroscience. 2014;**34**(4):1138-1147. DOI: 10.1523/JNEUROSCI.2852-13.2014

[68] Ross MH, Galaburda AM, Kemper TL. Down's syndrome: Is there a decreased population of neurons? Neurology. 1984;**34**:909-916. DOI: 10.1212/WNL.34.7.909

[69] Schmidt-Sidor B, Wisniewski KE, Shepard TH, Sersen EA. Brain growth in Down syndrome subjects 15 to 22 weeks of gestational age and birth to 60 months. Clinical Neuropathology. 1990;**9**:181-190

[70] Wisniewski KE. Down syndrome children often have brain with maturation delay, retardation of growth, and cortical dysgenesis. American Journal of Medical Genetics. 1990;**37**(Suppl 7):274-281. DOI: 10.1002/ajmg.1320370755

[71] Larsen KB, Laursen H, Graem N, Samuelsen GB, Bogdanovic N, et al. Reduced cell number in the neocortical part of the human fetal brain in Down syndrome. Annals of Anatomy. 2008;**190**:421-427. DOI: 10.1016/j.aanat.2008.05.007

[72] Golden JA, Hyman BT. Development of the superior temporal neocortex is anomalous in trisomy 21. Journal of Neuropathology and Experimental Neurology. 1994;**53**(5): 513-520. DOI: 10.1097/00005072-199409000-00011

Chapter 4

Sleep in Down Syndrome

Jasneek Chawla and Helen Heussler

Additional information is available at the end of the chapter

http://dx.doi.org/10.5772/intechopen.71065

Abstract

Sleep disorders are common, often overlooked problem in Down syndrome, particularly during childhood. Comorbidities such as congenital heart disease often present early and management of these needs to take priority. However, this can result in the lack of early development of good sleep habits and may also lead to the perception that sleep issues are an expected problem in children with Down syndrome, which do not require intervention. Studies have shown that sleep problems continue to be under-reported by parents of children with Down syndrome, even though conditions such as obstructive sleep apnoea are up to six times more common in this population. Therefore an understanding of the nature of sleep problems in Down syndrome is important for anyone working with this group. In this chapter we provide an overview of this topic, highlighting the key sleep issues encountered by children with Down syndrome, as well as providing a general approach to evaluation and management.

Keywords: Down syndrome, child, sleep, paediatrics

1. Introduction

Down syndrome (DS) or Trisomy 21 has an estimated prevalence ranging from 1/650 to 1/1000 live births [1–3], with over 270 affected babies born in Australia per year since 2007 [4]. It is the most common genetic cause of significant intellectual disability [5]. The condition is characterised by decline of IQ during infant and toddler years, well-documented impairments in the assimilation and expressive use of language, as well as in cognitive flexibility and memory [6]. Large inter-individual differences are seen within the DS population and numerous factors including genetics, epigenetics, early neural development and the environment are thought to have a role in how the DS phenotype expresses itself in each individual [7]. Variation in sleep patterns and sleep disruption, has been highlighted as another potential factor that could contribute to the wide phenotypic differences in DS; individuals with DS often have sleep fragmentation due to common co-existing sleep disorders [8–15]. The degree of sleep difficulties in an individual with DS may be important in determining their predisposition to cognitive decline, by contributing to pathological ageing [16].

2. Prevalence of sleep disorders in children with Down syndrome

Several clinical features of DS potentially lead to disturbed sleep and/or increased risk for sleep disordered breathing (SDB). However, not all of these characteristics are present in every child, and when present, vary in intensity [5]. Obstructive sleep apnoea (OSA) results from hypotonia, macroglossia and midface hypoplasia. Progressive obesity is an additional risk factor. Children with DS are also at increased risk for congenital heart disease, pulmonary hypertension, leukaemia, ear infections and scoliosis, [17] all comorbidities potentially associated with disrupted sleep [5].

Polysomnography (PSG) sleep studies undertaken in children with DS all suggest a much higher prevalence of OSA in children with DS compared to the 1–5% prevalence in the general paediatric population [18]. Studies estimate prevalence of OSA in children with DS ranging between 31 and 79% [8–10, 19, 20]. This wide range may be due to differences in study design; mean age of the children varied, with some groups using non-referred community-based samples [8, 9, 19, 20] and others including mixed groups with some participants who had been specifically referred with sleep concerns [10]. Individual groups also defined OSA differently, with some using higher cut-offs for apnoea-hypopnea (AHI) index than others. More accurate prevalence data comes from studies where the population has been better defined. Shott et al. [21] looked only at pre-school children with DS aged 2–4 years and found up to 80% had abnormal PSG results with 57% having evidence of OSA (defined as AHI >1/h). Others have shown that the prevalence of OSA remains high up to early school years [22]. Fitzgerald et al. [12] studied a referred sample of DS children who snored, reporting a mean AHI of 12.9/h, in 32/33 (97%) children. In the largest PSG study to date, Maris et al. [23] found a prevalence of OSA of 66.4% (AHI > 2.0/h) in 122 children with DS, with and without positive history for OSA, who underwent full overnight PSG. Importantly, even in those with a negative history for OSA, the prevalence was 53.8%. Regardless of the differences in study design, it is clear that the prevalence of OSA in children with DS is much higher than that in otherwise healthy children, being at least six times more common in DS.

Information regarding the prevalence of non-respiratory sleep difficulties in children with DS is obtained largely from questionnaire-based studies of parental report and is therefore subjective. Bedtime resistance, sleep anxiety, night waking, parasomnias and daytime sleepiness have all been reported commonly in children with DS [11, 13–15, 24]. Carter et al. [11] used the Child Sleep Habits Questionnaire (CSHQ) and found that parents universally reported sleep problems in school-aged children with DS that persisted into teenage years. Maris et al. [25] reported an overall prevalence of sleep problems of 74.1% in children with DS using the same questionnaire, with no correlation between sleep problems and underlying OSA. In a large email study of parents of children with DS, Rosen et al. [14] reported difficulties initiating sleep in 138/253 (51.8%) and difficulties maintaining sleep in 175/252 (69.4%) of children,

http://dx.doi.org/10.5772/intechopen.71065

with over half of the children (51.4%) described as having some degree of excessive daytime sleepiness. The response rate for this survey was only 46.5% from those contacted and therefore these results may not be truly representative of the entire population. However, similar findings have been shown by other groups [13].

3. Individual sleep disorders in children with Down syndrome

3.1. Obstructive sleep apnoea

Obstructive sleep apnoea (OSA) (**Figure 1**) refers to the presence of prolonged episodes of increased respiratory effort, associated with partial or complete upper airway obstruction and various combinations of snoring, intermittent hypoxia, hypercarbia, restless sleep, and increased number of awakenings [26]. Children with DS are anatomically at risk due to mid-facial and mandibular hypoplasia, relative macroglossia with a posterior tongue position, a shortened palate and narrowed nasopharynx. Hypotonia may also contribute to airway

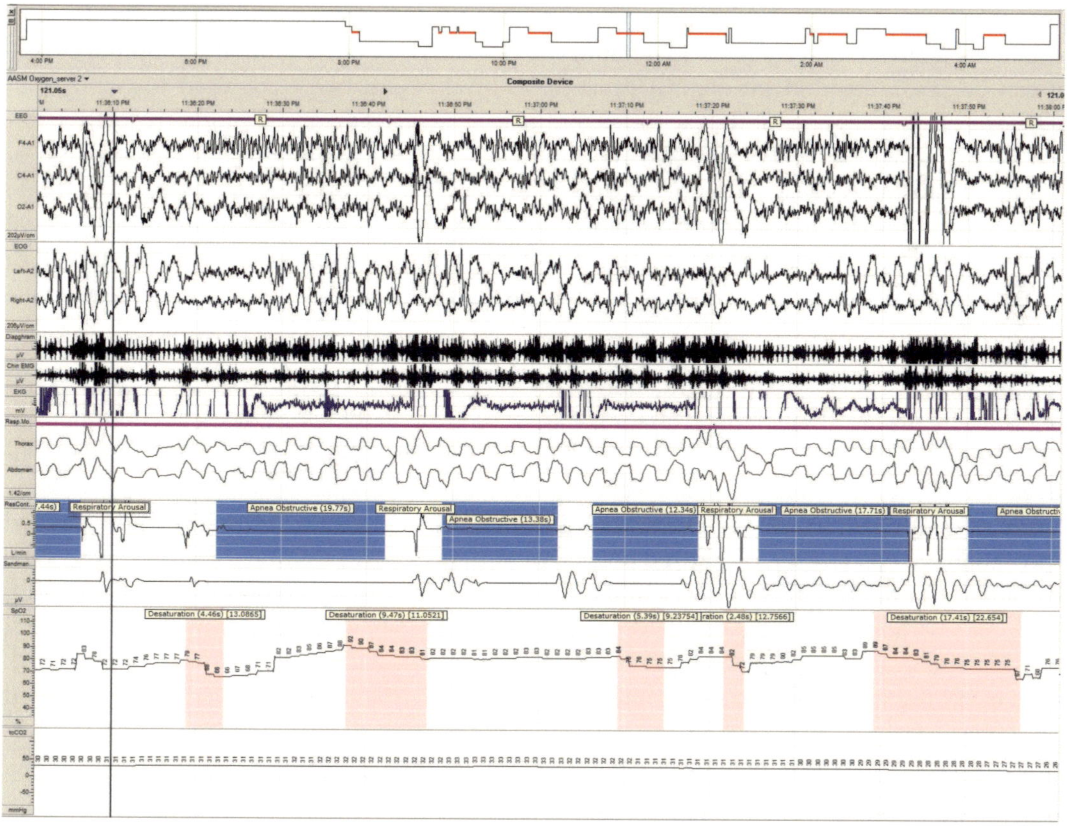

Figure 1. Diagnostic polysomnography (sleep study) recording demonstrating severe OSA-obstructive sleep apnoea in a 3 year old child with Down syndrome. Repetitive obstructive apnoeas are seen with absence of airflow but persisting and paradoxical respiratory effort. Associated respiratory arousals and oxygen desaturations (SpO2) are seen >3%.

collapse during sleep [27]. Lingual tonsil hypertrophy is also more common in DS with an 11-fold increase in incidence relative to typical controls [28]. Progressive obesity is an additional contributing risk factor and co-existing conditions such as gastro-oesophageal reflux disease, hypothyroidism and airway abnormalities such as laryngomalacia, subglottic and tracheal stenosis, which are more common in DS, may further exacerbate OSA [29]. Severity of OSA in DS often waxes and wanes, subsiding transiently through school age, due to growth and improved tone, but then reoccurring with onset of obesity in adolescent years.

International guidelines therefore recommend screening for OSA in children with DS [30, 31] but methods for screening are variable, largely due to available resources. The simplest method for screening is through clinical history from parental report. However, this often does not correlate with PSG findings; In their study of 65 children with DS, Shott et al. found that 69% of parents reported no sleep problems, yet 54% of these children had abnormal PSG [21]. Marcus et al. had similar results with only 32% of parents reporting clinical suspicion of OSA, despite a 100% incidence of abnormal study results [10].

Oximetry as a screening tool for OSA specifically in children with DS has had limited evaluation with conflicting results from available studies [32–34], which may be explained by differences in sample size. Increased sensitivity of oximetry to detect OSA may be possible through use of the McGill oximetry score [35] but further evaluation of this method is required before it can be recommended for clinical practice. Central events are recognised to occur with increased frequency in children with DS and may lead to difficulty with interpreting oximetry data [34] with respect to OSA. Similarly there may be more night-to-night variation of oximetry results in children with DS due to difficulties in achieving technically adequate monitoring [36]. Combined data from oximetry, parental report, actigraphy and audio-visual recording of sleep at home may overcome these difficulties, and provide a feasible method of screening for sleep disorders in children with DS [37].

At present, PSG (in-lab sleep study) remains the key investigation for diagnosis and quantification of OSA in DS. Sleep fragmentation, frequent awakenings and arousals and periodic leg movements are characteristic features described from early PSG studies in children with DS. These appear to occur with and without features of OSA [27]. Compared to controls, children with DS have been shown to have lower sleep efficiency and higher percentages of slow wave sleep (SWS) as well as reduced rapid eye movement (REM) sleep [38]. Mean oxygen saturation was also lower in children of all ages with DS and, in children aged 2–6.9 years the oxygen saturation nadir was lower in the DS subjects compared to controls. Another group have also demonstrated that children with OSA and DS had a similar symptom profile but slightly worse gas exchange than closely matched controls with OSA of similar severity [33]. This increased vulnerability to OSA may be partly due to the relative hypotonia and blunted cardiovascular responses seen in children with DS [39]. Congenital abnormalities in the pulmonary vasculature also increase the risk of pulmonary hypertension in DS [40].

Treatment of OSA in DS is not dissimilar to that in the TD population. Conservative measures such as weight loss and pharmacological treatments, including intranasal steroids or oral cysteinyl-leukotriene receptor antagonists (e.g. montelukast), can be tried in the first instance. Adenotonsillectomy (AT) remains the mainstay of treatment but has been shown to be associated with a higher respiratory complication rate [41] and appears to be less successful at treating the OSA in the DS population; Subjectively from parental report, Rosen et al. [14] found that out of 83 children with DS who had undergone AT, 38 (47.5%) continued to have witnessed apnoea and 22 (28.9%) continued to gasp and choke during sleep more than once a month. Objectively, three groups have shown that post AT, OAHI is reduced but does not fully normalise in this population, with approximately half of all children consistently shown to have a degree of residual OSA in all three studies [42–44]. All studies were however retrospective and included small numbers of patients. Two recent systematic reviews assessing outcomes post AT in DS children with OSA highlight the limited objective data available and also discuss some of the additional difficulties with drawing conclusions from existing evidence [45, 46]. The OAHI cut-offs taken to indicate benefit of surgery varies between studies and follow up times at which repeat PSG was performed also varied. It is also not clear from all studies whether repeat evaluation with PSG was performed in all patients post surgery or only those with residual symptoms which may introduce bias, with a paucity of data from those who may have improved. Nevertheless, despite these issues, the estimates of residual OSA have been reassuringly consistent and therefore cannot be entirely disregarded. In addition to the propensity for upper airway collapse and hypotonia, children with DS have multiple other comorbidities such as obesity and hypothyroidism, which likely contribute to the reasons why OSA persists in this group.

A variety of other surgical procedures including uvulopalatopharyngoplasty, lingual tonsillectomy, supraglottoplasty, partial midline glossectomy and tongue suspension with or without lingual tonsillectomy can be considered in children with persisting OSA post adenotonsillectomy. However, currently there is limited evidence to support the routine use of these procedures [47]. The benefit of these more aggressive surgical options for OSA specifically in the DS group is also unclear; Merrell and Shott [43] evaluated the use of lateral pharyngoplasty with adenotonsillectomy in the initial treatment of OSA in children with DS and found no additional benefit when compared to adenotonsillectomy alone. Wootten et al. [48] published their experience using combined genioglossus advancement and radiofrequency ablation of the tongue base in children with OSA refractory to AT. Successful treatment using this method (defined as a decrease in apnoea-hypopnea index, AHI, to <5/h on polysomnography, PSG) occurred in 12/19 patients with DS included in this study, suggesting this may be a promising option for future use but larger studies are required. The role of pre-evaluation of the airway with drug-induced sleep endoscopy (DISE) and cine magnetic resonance imaging (Cine-MRI) to direct surgical options for persistent OSA continues to undergo evaluation. However, these techniques have not yet been clearly linked to outcomes [47].Therefore, at present conservative treatment with continuous positive airway pressure (CPAP) or less commonly, bi-level (BPAP) therapy, is often preferred for management of residual OSA, preventing the need for further invasive surgical procedures including tracheostomy. Such therapy is however challenging in paediatrics and even more so in patients with DS, where behavioural and intellectual impairment may hinder the establishment and adherence to therapy. This may in particular apply to those children with comorbidity such as autism. Trois et al. [49] showed that in nine adults with DS who were prescribed CPAP, five had excellent compliance and experienced improvements in daytime functioning and excessive daytime sleepiness. Rosen [50] reported use of CPAP in three infants with DS and demonstrated spontaneous resolution of OSA after several months of use. Aside from this and early case reports, little has been published relating to CPAP use in the DS paediatric population.

3.2. Central sleep apnoea

Ferri et al. [51] 1st recognised the increased preponderance of central apnoeas (cessation of airflow and respiratory effort) in DS, which occurred in 89.4% of their patients (n = 10) irrespective of the presence of OSA (**Figure 2**). Coverstone et al. [34] reported that 32/119 (26.9%) children with DS had central apnoea indices ≥2.5/h on PSG, with 13 subjects (10%) having more central events than obstructive events. Another group found a prevalence of CSA (defined as central apnoea index CAI ≥1/h) of 41.6% in their study of 36 children with DS who underwent PSG evaluation [52]. In this study, AT for treatment of OSA resulted in resolution of CSA in 10 of these patients (66.7%). The mechanism behind this reduction was unclear and only a small number of children were included. Exactly what defines an abnormal CAI level in children, and particularly those with neurodevelopmental conditions, is unclear. Although a CAI > 1/h is by convention diagnostic of CSA, a CAI up to 5/h has been reported in healthy children up to the age of 13 years [53, 54]. Dysfunction of central respiratory control at a brainstem level

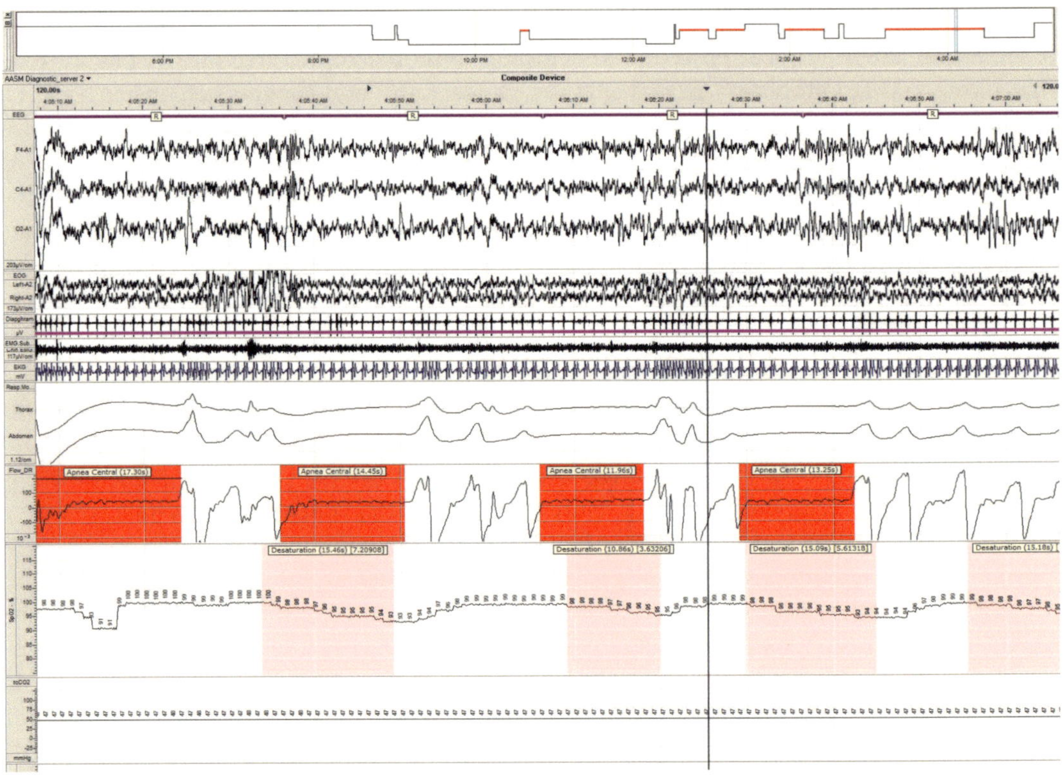

Figure 2. Diagnostic polysomnography (sleep study) recording demonstrating CSA-central sleep apnoea in a 6 year old child with Down syndrome. Repetitive central apnoeas are seen in a periodic breathing pattern, with absence of airflow and respiratory effort. Associated oxygen desaturations (SpO2) are seen >3%.

has been proposed as a potential aetiology for CSA in DS [51]. This could help to explain why there is an increased propensity for CSA in the very young DS group, who have immature respiratory control combined with hypotonia, which lessens over time [55]. Specific management and outcomes of CSA in DS have not been well described. A general approach would be to provide supplemental oxygen, with careful monitoring of carbon dioxide levels to ensure no increase occurs. Alternatively, if CSA is severe, non-invasvive ventilatory (NIV) support may be required to correct associated hypoxemia and hypoventilation with regular re-evaluation to monitor for spontaneous resolution of symptoms with age.

3.3. Non respiratory sleep disorders & circadian rhythm disorders

Studies have shown that bedtime resistance, sleep anxiety, night waking, parasomnias and daytime sleepiness are reported commonly in children with DS [11, 13–15]. These problems appear to begin at an early age and may continue to persist with increasing age. They also appear to persist despite treatment of OSA; Bassell et al. found that among 108 children with DS who had undergone AT for OSA, 55 (51%) continued to have sleep problems specifically in night awakenings, restless sleep, snoring and daytime sleepiness [56]. This would suggest that the sleep disruption seen in children with DS is not solely related to SDB, but is rather a feature of the condition itself. As seen with other disabilities, the child's intellectual limitation or communication problems may interfere with the acquisition of good sleep habits. Similarly the pressures associated with raising a child with developmental delay may impact parenting abilities, including the ability to cope with their child's sleep problems [57]. Comorbidities are also frequently described in children with DS and management of these can often take priority over the need to attend to sleep difficulties. Many of these can further exacerbate sleep problems either by increasing the risk for sleep disturbance in their own right, or by requiring the administration of medication that disrupts sleep continuity. The best example of this would be the use of stimulant drugs for attention-deficit-hyperactivity disorder (ADHD), a condition which has a high prevalence in children with DS [58].

Assessment of non-respiratory sleep disorders generally begins by obtaining a thorough sleep history from the child's main carer, gathering information on usual sleep habits and main areas of difficulty (e.g. difficulties with sleep onset through bedtime resistance or frequent night wakenings). Asking the parent/carer to keep a written sleep diary at home over a 1–2 week period, documenting the child's sleep over this time can be a useful way of gaining further details regarding usual routines.

Actigraphs, which are small movement detectors (accelerometers) placed on the child's wrist, can distinguish sleep from wake using algorithms to quantify the reduced movement associated with sleep. They have been shown to be a reliable method for determining sleep in children when compared against polysomnography (PSG) [59]. For clinical use the American Academy of Sleep Medicine recommends use of actigraphy for delineating sleep patterns and to document treatment responses in normal infants and children, and in special paediatric populations [60]. Objective data using actigraphy to assess sleep patterns in children with DS is limited. Chen et al. [61] found that children with disabilities in general experience difficulty with initiating sleep and maintaining sleep. However, the exact number of children with DS

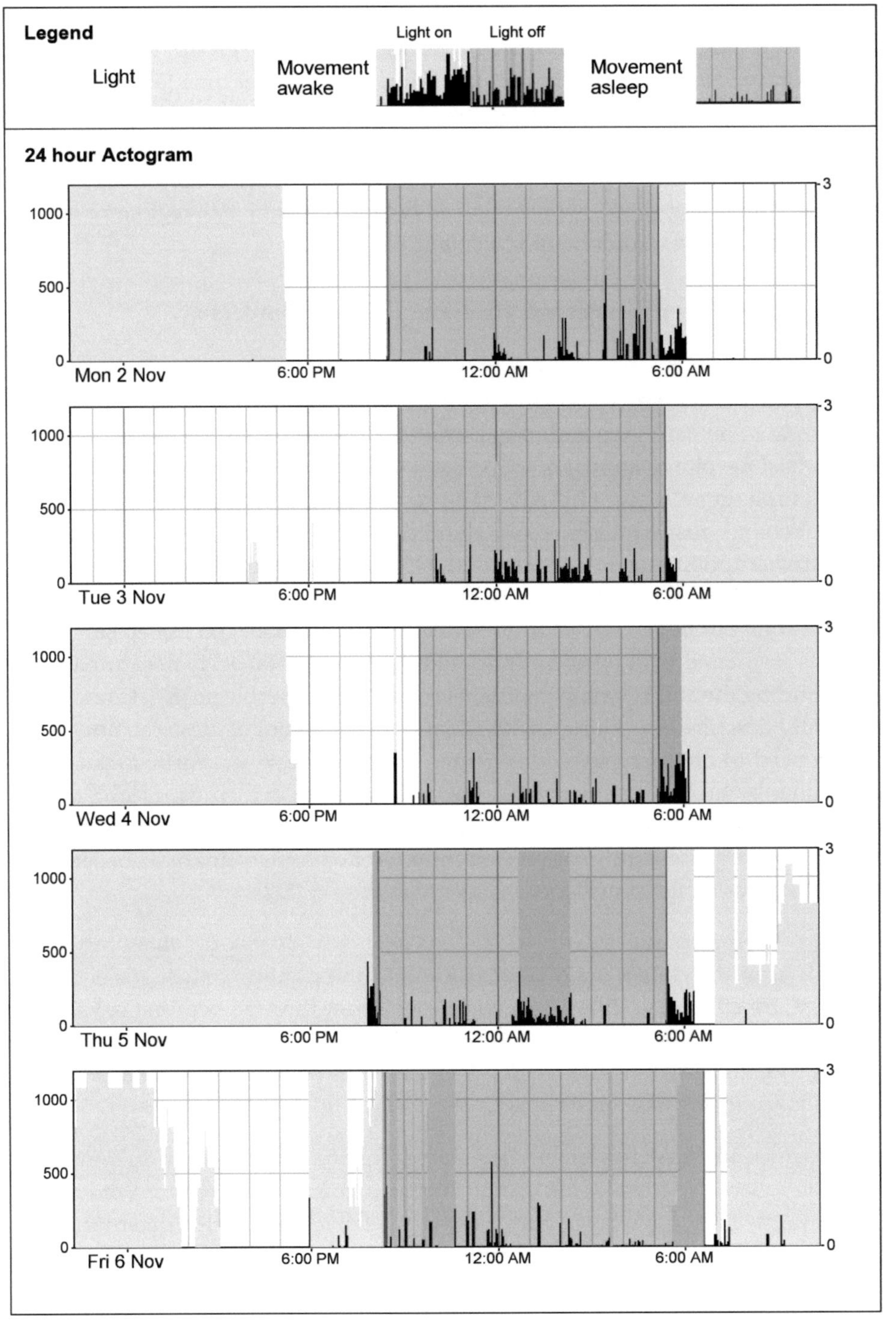

Figure 3. Example of how actigraphy demonstrates sleep-wake patterns recording shows variable sleep time, intermittent difficulty with sleep onset, restlessness and some overnight wakening.

http://dx.doi.org/10.5772/intechopen.71065

in this study is not clearly specified. Ashworth et al. [62] undertook a cross comparison of sleep problems in children with DS and Williams syndrome (WS) using actigraphy. Children with DS were found to have disrupted sleep, with considerably more night wakings, wake after sleep onset (WASO) and lower sleep efficiency than children with WS and TD controls. These studies suggest that actigraphy is feasible to undertake in children with DS and may be a useful tool to provide more objective data regarding sleep problems in this group in the future (**Figure 3**).

Several of the issues that lead to sleep difficulties in children with DS also present challenges in evaluation and management. Poor parental perception of sleep problems leads to under-reporting of these symptoms and therefore a lack of recognition and subsequent treatment by physicians. Due to the brain abnormalities present, sleep physiology and sleep-wake patterns may differ in this population resulting in children struggling to learn aspects of how and when to fall asleep. Studies investigating sleep and rhythm-related disturbances using mouse models of Down syndrome have consistently shown abnormal parameters but further study in human subjects is still required [63]. Psychological parental factors in this group likely impact on the ability to achieve a consistent, disciplined approach to their child's sleep pattern and to instil independent sleep habits [64]. Measures that are utilised in the TD such as parental education to encourage healthy sleep habits, behavioural interventions and selective use of pharmacological treatments such as melatonin can be used in children with DS. However, efficacy studies assessing response are limited in this group and success is likely to be dependent on parental capabilities and commitment, as well as the child's willingness and ability to comply [57].

Therefore currently, treatment options for non-respiratory sleep disorders in children with DS are not dissimilar to those for the TD. Good sleep hygiene as defined by routine, clear expectations and limit setting, self-calming strategies and management of light/dark are key to successful implementation of sleep initiation and scheduling challenges.

4. Potential impact of sleep disorders in children with Down syndrome

The adverse effects of poor sleep are increasingly recognised with studies in TD children describing substantial morbidities affecting the central nervous system (CNS), cardiovascular, metabolic systems and somatic growth, ultimately leading to reduced quality of life [65]. Children with DS are more vulnerable to these complications as they are already at high risk for some of these conditions. For example, infants with DS have been shown to have a higher prevalence of pulmonary hypertension [40], which is also associated with OSA in patients with DS [66] and therefore cardiovascular complications of OSA are likely to be even more dangerous in patients with DS as compared with patients without DS [29].

Of particular relevance to the DS population is the mounting evidence in TD children regarding the negative impact of sleep deprivation [67] and SDB [68–73] on cognition, behaviour and academic performance. Sleep disruption in children with neurodevelopmental disorders may exacerbate learning difficulties and disturbed behaviour that are part of the developmental disorder itself [38]. The high prevalence of sleep disorders during childhood may make children with DS particularly susceptible to ill effects during critical periods of cognitive development. Small cross sectional studies have found deficits in IQ [6], cognitive and behavioural function [74–77] and accomplishment of daily activities [78] in children with DS and co-existing sleep problems, suggesting an association between poor sleep and these deficits in this group. The age range evaluated in these studies has varied with some groups concentrating on pre-school children with DS [75–77] and others examining older children [6, 74, 78]. All the studies evaluating cognition and behaviour include very small numbers of children with the largest being an un-referred community sample of 38 individuals. The differences in study design used by each group makes it difficult to combine findings from these small reports for meta-analysis, with the major difficulty being the different measures used by each group. Some have used formal assessment with PSG or cardiorespiratory polygraphy to identify sleep problems, focusing primarily on the presence of SDB, whereas others have relied on questionnaire-based parental reports of broad sleep problems, primarily using the Child Sleep Habits Questionnaire (CSHQ). The cognitive and behavioural outcomes evaluated have also differed greatly with some groups undertaking batteries of tests examining various different aspects of cognitive and behaviour performance and others concentrating on a specific area, such as executive function or language. Three groups clearly stated that the participants were from community samples whereas in other studies this was not clearly defined. Control groups of TD children for comparison were included in some designs but not others. Despite this heterogeneity in study methodology, results do consistently suggest an association between sleep and cognitive and behavioural outcomes. Two studies have examined inter-group differences; comparing DS children with sleep and without sleep problems. Breslin et al. [6] compared 19 children with DS and comorbid OSA on PSG (AHI > 1.5/h) with 12 children with DS and no OSA. This study convincingly demonstrated worse outcomes in the OSA group with a 9-point difference in Verbal IQ and impairments in cognitive flexibility in children with DS and comorbid OSA, compared to those without OSA. Edgin et al. [75] divided their group of pre-school children with DS into poor sleepers (DS PS) and good sleepers (DS GS) using actigraphy data and compared them to each other, as well as to TD controls, assessing language skills and behaviour. Strikingly they found that only 31.6% of children with DS in the PS group were combining words, as compared to 80% of good sleepers. Additionally poorer language was shown to relate to the level of sleep disruption.

Only one group has assessed the association between sleep and functional ability in children with DS. Churchill et al. [78] conducted a large internet based cross sectional survey study which included 110 parents of children with DS and 29 parents of children with TD aged 5–18 years. They found that sleep disturbances, assessed with the CSHQ, were negatively related to accomplishment of daily life functions described using the Life Habit questionnaire (Life-H). This finding is an important one as it suggests that sleep disorders in this population have significant impact of daily life and this has wider implications on how these children may function later in life. As the authors point out, the unanswered question is whether treating sleep problems in children with DS leads to improved accomplishment of daily life habits and other important life outcomes. Further work in this area is necessary as improved understanding of the interaction between sleep and functional outcomes in this group may lead to

http://dx.doi.org/10.5772/intechopen.71065

significant long-term benefits for these children. It may also help to inform researchers who are currently working to understand the role of poor sleep and increased risk of development of Alzheimer's disease seen in adult patients with DS.

5. Summary

Understanding that children with DS are high risk for a variety of common sleep problems and the potential impact of this on both the child and their family is essential for health professionals working with this population. Existing international guidelines recommend regular screening for sleep problems as part of routine clinical care for children with DS [30, 31]. However resources for sleep evaluation are limited and an awareness of the potential negative impact of untreated sleep problems in this population is lacking among both clinicians and parents. Currently there is wide variation in practice relating to this area, with often the perception that these problems can be ignored and left untreated in children with DS as these children already have established intellectual disability. The fact that treatment is often more challenging in DS compared to TD children can also contribute to the lack of attempt to treat sleep disorders in this group. Treatment options are similar to those in TD children but have less successful outcomes. In particular many children are left with residual OSA, highlighting the need for further evaluation of strategies that may improve toleration of conservative measures such as CPAP therapy, as well as exploring newer surgical options to determine specific benefit in this population. Other areas of future research include improving the understanding of the link between poor sleep and long-term outcomes in children with DS, which may assist in improving quality of life and independence for this population, through earlier treatment of sleep difficulties using specifically tailored sleep programmes.

Author details

Jasneek Chawla[1,3,4]* and Helen Heussler[1,2,3,4]

*Address all correspondence to: Jasneek.chawla@health.qld.gov.au

1 Paediatric Respiratory & Sleep Medicine, Lady Cilento Children's Hospital, Brisbane, Australia

2 Child Development, Lady Cilento Children's Hospital, Brisbane, Australia

3 School of Medicine, The University of Queensland, Brisbane, Australia

4 Mater Medical Research Institute, The University of Queensland, Brisbane, Australia

References

[1] Irving C, Basu A, Richmond S, Burn J, Wren C. Twenty-year trends in prevalence and survival of Down syndrome. European Journal of Human Genetics. 2008;**16**:1336-1340

[2] Sherman S, Allen EG, Bean LH, Freeman SB. Epidemiology of Down syndrome. Mental Retardation and Developmental Disabilities Research Reviews. 2007;**13**:221-227

[3] Sommer C, Henrique-Silva F. Trisomy 21 and Down syndrome: A short review. Brazilian Journal of Biology. 2008;**68**:447-452

[4] Down Syndrome Australia. Available from: https://www.downsyndrome.org.au/research_and_statistics.html#statistics

[5] Churchill S, Kieckhefer GM, Landis CA, Ward TM. Sleep measurement and monitoring in children with Down syndrome: A review of the literature, 1960-2010. Sleep Medicine Reviews. 2012;**16**(5):477-488

[6] Breslin J, Spano G, Bootzin R, Anand P, Nadel L, Edgin J. Obstructive sleep apnea syndrome and cognition in Down Syndrome. Developmental Medicine and Child Neurology. 2014;**56**(7):657-664

[7] Karmiloff-Smith A, Al-Janabi T, D'Souza H, Groet J, Massand E, Mok K, et al. The importance of understanding indivdiual differences in Down syndrome. F1000 Research. 2016;**5**(F1000 Faculty Rev):389

[8] Dyken M, Lin-Dyken DC, Poulton S, Zimmerman MB, Sedars E. Prospective polysomnographic analysis of obstructive sleep apnea in Down syndrome. Archives of Pediatrics & Adolescent Medicine. 2003;**157**:655-660

[9] Ng D, Hui HN, Chan CH, Kwok KL, Chow PY, Cheung JM, et al. Obstructive sleep apnoea in children with Down syndrome. Singapore Medical Journal. 2006;**47**(9):774-779

[10] Marcus C, Keens TG, Bautista DB, von Pechmann WS, Ward SLD. Obstructive sleep apnea in children with Down Syndrome. Pediatrics. 1991;**88**(1):132-139

[11] Carter M, McCaughey E, Annaz D, Hill CM. Sleep problems in a Down syndrome population. Archives of Disease in Childhood. 2009;**94**:308-310

[12] Fitzgerald D, Paul A, Richmond C. Severity of obstructive apnoea in children with Down syndrome who snore. Archives of Disease in Childhood. 2007;**92**(5):423

[13] Hoffmire C, Magyar CI, Connolly HV, Fernandez D, van Wijngaarden E. High prevalence of sleep disorders and associated comorbidities in a community sample of children with Down syndrome. Journal of Clinical Sleep Medicine. 2014;**10**(4):411-419

[14] Rosen D, Lombardo A, Skotko B, Davidson EJ. Parental perceptions of sleep disturbances and sleep disordered breathing in children with Down syndrome. Clinical Pediatrics. 2011;**50**(2):121-125

[15] Breslin J, Edgin JO, Bootzin RR, Goodwin JL, Nadel L. Parental report of sleep problems in Down syndrome. Journal of Intellectual Disability Research. 2011;**55**(11):1086-1091

[16] Fernandez F, Edgin J. Poor sleep as a precursor to cognitive decline in Down syndrome: A hypothesis. Journal of Alzheimers Disease and Parkinsonism. 2013;**3**(2):124

[17] Bittles A, Bower C, Hussain R, Glasson EJ. The four ages of Down syndrome. European Journal of Public Health. 2006;**17**(2):221-225

[18] Marcus C, Brooks LJ, et al. Diagnosis and management of childhood obstructive sleep apnea syndrome. Clinical Report Pediatrics. 2012;**130**:576-584

[19] de Miguel-Diez J, Villa-Asensi, JR., Alvarez-Sala, JL. Prevalence of sleep-disordered breathing in children with Down syndrome: Polygraphic findings in 108 children. Sleep 2003;**26**(8):1006-1009

[20] Stebbens V, Dennis J, Samuels MP, Croft CB, Southall DP. Sleep related upper airway obstruction in a cohort with Down's syndrome Arch Dis in. Childhood. 1991;**66**:1333-1338

[21] Shott S, Amin R, Chini B, Heubi C, Hotze S, Akers R. Obstructive sleep apnea: Should all children with Down syndrome be tested? Archives of Otolaryngology – Head & Neck Surgery. 2006;**132**(4):432-436

[22] Austeng M, Øverland B, Kværner KJ, Andersson EM, Axelsson S, Abdelnoor M, et al. Obstructive sleep apnea in younger school children with Down syndrome. International Journal of Pediatric Otorhinolaryngology. 2014;**78**:1026-1029

[23] Maris M, Verhulst S, Woiciechowski M, Van de Heyning P, Boudewyns A. Prevalence of obstructive sleep apnea in children with Down syndrome. Sleep. 2016;**39**(3):699-704

[24] Cotton S, Richdale A. Brief report: Parental descriptions if sleep problems in children with autism, Down syndrome and Prader-Willi syndrome. Research in Developmental Disabilities. 2006;**27**:151-161

[25] Maris M, Verhulst S, Woiciechowski M, Van de Heyning P, Boudewyns A. Sleep problems and obstructive sleep apnoea in children with Down syndrome, an overview. International Journal of Pediatric Otorhinolaryngology. 2016;**82**:12-15

[26] American Academy of Sleep Medicine. International Classification of Sleep Disorders. Diagnostic and Coding Manual. 2nd ed. Westchester IL; 2005

[27] Levanon A, Tarasiuk A, Tal A. Sleep characteristics in children with Down syndrome. The Journal of Pediatrics. 1999;**134**:755-760

[28] Fricke B, Donnelly LF, Shott SR, Kalra M, Poe SA, Chini BA, et al. Comparison of lingual tonsil size as depicted on MR imaging between children with obstructive sleep apnea despite previous tonsillectomy and adenoidectomy and normal controls. Pediatric Radiology. 2006;**36**(6):518-523

[29] Lal C, White DR, Joseph JE, van Bakergem K, LaRosa A. Sleep-disordered breathing in Down syndrome. Chest 2015;**147**(2):570-579

[30] Working party on sleep physiology and respiratory control disorders in children. Standards of Services for Children with Disorders of Sleep Physiology Report. Royal College of Paediatrics and Child Health. 2009

[31] Bull M, the Committee on Genetics. Health supervision for children with Down syndrome. Pediatrics. 2011;**128**(2):393-406

[32] Jheeta S, McGowan M, Hadjikoumi I. Is oximetry an effective screening tool for obstructive sleep apnoea in children with Down syndrome? Archives of Disease in Childhood. 2013;**98**:164

[33] Lin S, Davey MJ, Horne RS, Nixon GM. Screening of obstructive sleep apnea in children with Down syndrome. The Journal of Pediatrics. 2014;**165**(1):117-122

[34] Coverstone A, Bird M, Sicard M, Tao Y, Grange DK, Cleveland C, et al. Overnight pulse oximetry for evaluation of sleep apnea among children with trisomy 21. Journal of Clinical Sleep Medicine. 2014;**10**(12):1309-1315

[35] Brouillette R, Morielli A, Leimanis A, Waters KA, et al. Nocturnal pulse oximetry as an abbreviated testing modality for pediatric obstructive sleep apnea. Pediatrics. 2000;**105**(2):405-412

[36] Burke R, Maxwell B, Hunter C, Graham D, O'Donoghue D, Shields M. Night-tonight variation of pulse oximetry in children with sleep disordered breathing. Archives of Disease in Childhood. 2016;**101**:1095-1099

[37] Stores R, Stores G. The significance of aspects of screening for obstructive sleep apnoea in children with Down syndrome. Journal of Intellectual Disability Research. 2014;**58**(4): 381-392

[38] Nisbet L, Phillips NN, Hoban TF, O'Brien LM. Characterization of a sleep architectural phenotype in children with Down syndrome. Sleep & Breathing. 2015;**19**:1065-1071

[39] O'Driscoll D, Horne RSC, Davey MJ, Hope SA, Anderson V, Trinder J, et al. Cardiac and sympathetic activation are reduced in children with Down syndrome and sleep disordered breathing. Sleep. 2012;**35**(9):1269-1275

[40] Cua L, Blankenship A, North AL, Hayes J, Nelin LD. Increased incidence of idiopathic persistent pulmonary hypertension in Down syndrome neonates. Pediatric Cardiology. 2007;**28**(4):250-254

[41] Goldstein N, Armfield DR, Kingsley LA, Borland LM, Allen GC, Post JC. Postoperative complications after tonsillectomy and adenoidectomy in children with Down syndrome. Archives of Otolaryngology – Head & Neck Surgery. 1998;**124**(2):171-176

[42] Shete M, Stocks RMS, Sebelik ME, Schoumacher RA. Effects of adeno-tonsillectomy on polysomnography patterns in Down syndrome children with obstructive sleep apnea: A comparative study with children without Down syndrome. International Journal of Pediatric Otorhinolaryngology. 2010;**74**:241-244

[43] Merrell JS, Shott SR. OSAS in Down syndrome: T&A versus T&A plus lateral pharyngoplasty. International Journal of Pediatric Otorhinolaryngology. 2007;**71**:1197-1203

[44] Maris M, Verhulst S, Woiciechowski M, Van de Heyning P, Boudewyns A. Outcome of adentonsillectomy in children with Down syndrome and obstructive sleep apnoea. Archives of Disease in Childhood. 2016. DOI: 10.1136/archdischild-2015-310351 [Epub ahead of print]

[45] Farhood Z, Isley JW, Ong A, Nguyen SA, Camilon TJ, LaRosa AC, et al. Adenotonsillectomy outcomes in patients with Down syndrome and obstructive sleep apnea. The Laryngoscope. 2017;**127**(6):1465-1470

[46] Nation J, Brigger M. The efficacy of adenotonsillectomy for obstructive sleep apnea in children with Down syndrome: A systematic review. Otolaryngology and Head and Neck Surgery. 2017

[47] Manickam P, Shott SR, Boss EF, Cohen AP, Meinzen-Derr JK, Amin RS, Ishman SL. Systematic review of site of obstruction identification and non-CPAP treatment options for children with persistent paediatric obstructive sleep apnea. The Laryngoscope. 2015;**126**:491-500

[48] Wootten CS, Shott SR. Evolving therapties to treat retroglossal and base-of-tongue obstruction in pediatric obstructive sleep apnea. Archives of Otolaryngology – Head & Neck Surgery. 2010;**136**(10):983-987

[49] Trois M, Capone GT, Lutz JA, Melendres MC, Schwartz AR, Collop NA, et al. Obstructive sleep apnea in adults with Down syndrome. Journal of Clinical Sleep Medicine. 2009;**5**(4):317-323

[50] Rosen D. Some infants with Down syndrome spontaneously outgrow their obstructive sleep apnea. Clinical Pediatrics. 2010;**49**(11):1068-1071

[51] Ferri R, Curzi-Dascalova L, Del Gracco S, Elia M, Musumeci SA, Stefanini MC. Respiratory patterns during sleep in Down's syndrome: Importance of central apnoeas. Journal of Sleep Research. 1997;**6**:134-141

[52] Thottam P, Choi S, Simons JP, Kitsko DO. Effect of adenotonsillectomy on central and obstructive sleep apnea in children with Down syndrome. Otolaryngology and Head and Neck Surgery. 2015;**153**(4):644-648

[53] Felix O, Amaddeo A, Arroyo JO, Zerah M, Puget S, Cormier-Daire V, et al. Central sleep apnea in children: Experience at a single center. Sleep Medicine. 2016;**25**:24-28

[54] Kritzinger F, Al-Saleh S, Narang I. Descriptive analysis of central sleep apnea in childhood at a single center. Pediatric Pulmonology. 2011;**46**:1023-1030

[55] Fan Z, Ahn M, Roth HL, Li L, Vaughn BV. Sleep apnea and hypoventilation in patients with Down syndrome: Analysis of 144 polysomnogram studies. Children. 2017;**4**(7):55 DOI:10.3390/children4070055 (online first)

[56] Bassell J, Phan H, Leu R, Kronk R, Visootsak J. Sleep profiles in children with Down syndrome. American Journal of Medical Genetics Part A. 2015;**167A**:1830-1835

[57] Stores G, Stores R. Sleep disorders and their clinical significant in children with Down syndrome. Developmental Medicine and Child Neurology. 2012;**55**:126-130

[58] Ekstein S, Glick B, Weill M, Kay B, Berger I. Down syndrome and attention-deficit/hyperactivity disorder (ADHD). Journal of Child Neurology. 2011;**26**(10):1290-1295

[59] Hyde M, O'Driscoll DM, Binette S, Galang C, Tan SK, Verginis N, et al. Validation of actigraphy for deterining sleep and wake in children with sleep disordered breathing. Journal of Sleep Research. 2007;**16**:213-216

[60] Morgenthaler T, Alessi C, Friedman L, Owens J, Kapur V, Boehlecke B, et al. Practice parameters for the use of actigraphy in the assessment of sleep and sleep disorders: An update for 2007. Sleep. 2007;**30**(4):519-529

[61] Chen X, Velez JC, Barbosa C, Pepper M, Gelaye B, Redline S, et al. Evaluation of actigraphy-measured sleep patterns among children with disabilities and associations with caregivers' educational attainment: Results from a cross-sectional study. BMJ Open. 2015;**5**(12):e008589

[62] Ashworth A, Hill CM, Karmiloff-Smith A, Dimitriou D. Cross syndrome comparison of sleep problems in children with Down syndrome and Williams syndrome. Research in Developmental Disabilities. 2013;**34**:1572-1580

[63] Heise I, Fisher SP, Banks GT, Wells S, Peirson SN, Foster RG, et al. Sleep-like behavior and 24-h rhythm disruption in the Tc1 mouse model of Down syndrome Genes. Brain and Behavior. 2015;**14**:209-216

[64] Richdale A, Wiggs L. Behavioural approaches to the treatment of sleep problems in children with developmental disorders: What is state of the art? International Journal of Behavioral and Consultation Therapy. 2005;**1**(3):165-188

[65] Capdevila OS, Kheirandish-Gozal L, Dayyat E, Gozal D. Paediatric obstructive sleep apnea complications, management and long-term outcomes. Proceedings of the American Thoracic Society. 2008;**5**:274-282

[66] Loughlin GM, Wynne JW, Victorica BE. Sleep apnea as a possible cause of pulmonary hypertension in Down syndrome. The Journal of Pediatrics. 1981;**98**(3):435-437

[67] Maski K, Kothare SV. Sleep deprivation and neurobehavioral functioning in children. International Journal of Psychophysiology. 2013;**89**(2):259-264

[68] Beebe DW. Neurobehavioural morbidity associated with disordered breathing in sleep in children: A comprehensive review. Sleep. 2006;**29**:1115-1134

[69] Blunden S, Lushington K, Lorenzen B, et al. Neuropsychological and psychosocial function in children with a history of snoring or behavioural problems. The Journal of Pediatrics. 2005;**146**(6):780

[70] Blunden SLK, Lorenzen B, Martin J, Kennedy D. Behavior and neurocognitive performance in children aged 5-10 years who snore compared to controls. Journal of Clinical and Experimental Neuropsychology. 2000;**22**(5):554-568

[71] Bourke R, Anderson V, Yang J, et al. Cognitive and academic functions are impaired in children with all severities of sleep-disordered breathing. Sleep Medicine. 2011;**12**:489-496

[72] Bourke R, Anderson V, Yang J, et al. Neurobehavioural function is impaired in children with all severities of sleep disordered breathing. Sleep Medicine. 2011;**12**:222-229

[73] Marcus C, Moore R, Rosen C, et al. A randomized trial of adenotonsillectomy for childhood sleep apnea. New England Journal of Medicine. 2013;**368**:2366-2376

[74] Chen C, Spano G, Edgin JO. The impact of sleep disruption on executive function in Down syndrome. Research in Developmental Disabilities. 2013;**34**(6):2033-2039

[75] Edgin J, Tooley U, Demara B, Nyhuis C, Anand P, Spano G. Sleep disturbance and expressive language development in preschool-age children with Down syndrome. Child Development. 2015;**86**(6):1984-1998

[76] Joyce A, Dimitriou D. Sleep-disordered breathing and cognitive functioning in preschool children with and without Down syndrome. Journal of Intellectual Disability Research. 2017;Jun 14 [Epub ahead of print]

[77] Lukowski A, Milojevich HM. Sleep problems and temperament in young children with Down syndrome and typically develping controls. Journal of Intellectual Disability Research. 2017;**61**(3):221-232

[78] Churchill S, Kieckhefer GM, Bjornson KF, Herting JR. Relationship between sleep disturbance and functional outcomes in daily life habits of children with Down syndrome. Sleep. 2015;**38**(1):61-71

Section 3

Prenatal Diagnosis

Chapter 5

Prenatal Diagnosis of Down Syndrome

Iliescu Dominic-Gabriel and
Drăgușin Roxana-Cristina

Additional information is available at the end of the chapter

http://dx.doi.org/10.5772/intechopen.71064

Abstract

The chapter's contribution to the book explores the prenatal modalities to diagnose Down syndrome (DS). The current knowledge in the field of genetic sonographic markers is presented, along the performance of current policies as well as the potential of new emerging genetic techniques. Besides the screening or testing pregnancy algorithms, the chapter describes the power of prenatal diagnostic techniques, namely, the advantages and the complications of the invasive genetic maneuvers. The progress in prenatal diagnosis of Down syndrome is one of the most important in prenatal medicine in the last decades. The methods vary in terms of detection rates, acceptability, costs, and potential complications. Although the early genetic screening was improved, ultrasound evaluation should not be dismissed, as the first-trimester sonography has the potential to diagnose the majority of major fetal abnormalities.

Keywords: Down syndrome, prenatal diagnosis, ultrasound, first trimester, nuchal translucency, nasal bone, facial angle, cell-free DNA, combined test, genetic ultrasonogram

1. Introduction

More than 1 in 1000 newborns is affected by Down syndrome (DS) [1], a disease that necessitates significant societal financial and legal support, because about 85% of infants survive the first year and 50% of those will live longer than 50 years [2]. As aneuploidies are major causes of perinatal death and childhood handicap, screening for fetal chromosomal abnormalities should be available to all pregnant women as an essential part of antenatal care and comprehensive counseling.

Fortunately, DS can be suspected during pregnancy by combined ultrasound and serologic screening and confirmed by invasive genetic techniques [3]. Also, genetic noninvasive tests were recently developed that reach near certitude detection rates. First-trimester detection of fetal major abnormalities, including trisomy 21, is important, because it offers the couples the advantages of early termination of pregnancy: less medical complications, reduced economical costs to the health system, and minor emotional impact of the couple. And we should keep in mind that the abortion rates in DS-affected pregnancies have increased to 67–92% in the United States and Europe [4].

Today, the screening methods for trisomy 21 fetuses are multiple, and patients need to choose early and comfortable. All pregnant women should be offered screening for aneuploidies, even if not all patients will accept. The expertise of a genetics counselor, preconceptual or in the first trimester, is beneficial for comprehensive counseling.

2. Historical aspects of aneuploidy screening: evolution and efficiency

The prenatal screening for chromosomal abnormalities was traditionally addressed to DS [5], because this is the most common chromosomal disease in fetuses and accounts for 8% of all congenital abnormal newborns.

It is well known that the chance of having a child with this condition increases as a woman gets older [6, 7], thus, in the 1970s and many decades after, maternal age represented the main screening method for fetal aneuploidy, by offering the option of genetic amniocentesis to all pregnant women over 35 years [8]. In the 1980s, determination of maternal serum alpha-fetoprotein (AFP) was proposed for screening, as decreased levels associated with an increased risk for DS [9]. During the last decades, diagnostic ultrasonography in obstetrics had a dramatic impact in prenatal medicine care, providing valuable information regarding fetal physiology, development, and abnormal conditions, including markers for fetal aneuploidies since the early 1990s [10, 11]. Human chorionic-gonadotrophin (HCG) and unconjugated estriol (uE3) testing were added along AFP determination, resulting in the serology triple test screen [12], and the detection rates were reported up to 73%, in the early 1990s [13]. The quad test was introduced after 1996, by including inhibin-A as a fourth marker to the triple test with a sensitivity of 81% at a 5% screen-positive rate [14, 15]. Also, during the 1990s, Kypros Nicolaides identified a powerful ultrasound marker measurable in the first trimester, namely, increased nuchal translucency (NT) thickness [16]. A first-trimester scan, also named nuchal scan or the genetic scan, was proposed as method for screening of major aneuploidies in combination with maternal age and serum testing (beta human chorionic gonadotropin (beta HCG) and pregnancy-associated plasma protein-A (PAPP-A)). Increased nuchal translucency, reduced PAPP-A levels, and an increased HCG are associated with a higher risk for DS, and using specific calculators, these ultrasound and serologic parameters assist practitioners in identifying pregnancies at risk, by using specific calculators, as the software developed by The Fetal Medicine Foundation [17, 18]. The detection rates for trisomy 21 were reported as 70–82% for first-trimester NT and 87% for first-trimester NT and serum. Additional evaluation of several ultrasound markers increases the detection rate to 90%, when the nasal bone is screened, and 95% with supplementary assessment of the blood flow through the tricuspid valve and ductus venosus (DV), which is similar to the technique that combines first-trimester NT and serum and second-trimester serologic QUAD test [19].

3. Strategies to perform aneuploidy screening

Current guidelines state that every pregnant woman of all ages should be offered extensive genetic counseling, screening, and invasive diagnostic testing for pregnancy with increased genetic risk before 20-week gestation [20]. Pregnant women should decide the genetic investigation technique after extensive counseling regarding the advantages, limitations, the sensibility, and false-positive results of every genetic test available [21, 22]. Still, because of limited healthcare system resources, the present screening options in the first trimester include nuchal translucency testing in combination with measurement of PAPP-A and HCG. In the second trimester, the screening tests include serum screening using triple or quadruple screening and ultrasonography. There is also the possibility for combination of first- and second-trimester screening in an integrated, stepwise sequential, or contingent sequential fashion [20, 23, 24]. Recently, some professional societies adopted the noninvasive cell-free fetal DNA in the detection protocol, for the cases with intermediate-risk cases. This relatively new test will be described separately in the chapter.

3.1. First-trimester markers and further benefit for pregnancy screening

Using only NT testing, the DS detection rate is only approximately 70% for a 5% false-positive rate [25]. However, an increased nuchal translucency greater than 3.5 mm is associated not only with genetic syndromes but also with fetal malformations, as major congenital heart defects, skeletal dysplasia, and congenital diaphragmatic hernia; thus, this marker is important for early detection of such structural abnormalities.

The first-trimester maternal serum screening includes the determination of two markers, PAPP-A and HCG. PAPP-A is a glycoprotein [26] produced by the placental syncytiotrophoblast and decidua that is decreased when placental function is abnormal, as reported in many aneuploidies and other pregnancy complications, as miscarriage and fetal growth restriction [27]. High levels of the HCG glycoprotein are usually present in DS pregnancies [28], and low levels of both markers are also associated with adverse pregnancy outcomes, such as miscarriage, stillbirth, preeclampsia, placental abruption, preterm birth, and low birth weight [29]. The serum concentration of these markers is converted to multiples of median (MoMs) and interpreted in combination with NT MoM and maternal age by dedicated software [30, 31]. The result of this combined test estimates the pregnancy genetic risk, which is considered low or increased, using a cutoff of 1/250. There are several strategies to define an intermediate risk, for example, from 1/50 or 1/100 to 1/1000. The risk in this population may be further refined with the aid of other ultrasound markers (nasal bone, tricuspid valve, and ductus venosus blood flow) or second-trimester markers, as a contingent or sequential approach [19]. More recently, the use of cell-free fetal DNA is advocated and implemented in some healthcare systems (England, Denmark, and Holland).

There are several strategies regarding the timing of the ultrasound and serological determinations. For best patient compliance, OSCAR method is preferred (one-step assessment of risk)—with biological and ultrasound evaluations, result, and parent counseling performed in one session. However, a 2–4% improvement of the detection rate is obtained, if screening is carried in two separate visits, with maternal serum testing at 9–10 weeks of gestation (when the determinations are more specific) and the ultrasound scan at 12 weeks (for a better visualization of fetal anatomy) [32, 33]. Laboratory certification and periodically sonographer audit are important, due to the necessity of precise measurements [22].

3.2. Second-trimester screening strategies

The second-trimester maternal serum testing includes the triple and quadruple screens, with detection rates of 70 and 81%, respectively [22].

As in the first trimester, the ultrasound scan can be used for screening either alone or as an adjunct to maternal serum testing. Various sonographic features were proposed as markers for fetal chromosomal abnormalities [34, 35], and a 75% detection rate was reported for second-trimester genetic ultrasonography [36].

First- and second-trimester screening data can be combined to improve the detection or to lower the false-positive rate to 5% [37]. *Integrated* screening involves a unitary report of first-trimester combined test, followed by triple or quadruple screen in the second trimester. *Stepwise sequential* strategy allows the patients at increased risk to opt for invasive diagnostic testing or to await the second-trimester screen to revise the genetic risk. The *contingency* screening is based on a stratified risk determination in the first trimester. In high-risk pregnancy, invasive diagnostic testing is offered; in low-risk patients, no further testing is required; and in intermediate group, between the two cutoffs, second-trimester screening is advised [14].

Fetal echocardiography, even if difficult to apply as a primary screening tool, can be comparable to first-trimester integrated screening in identifying over 90% of fetuses with trisomy 21 [19]. Still, it can be used after 20 weeks of gestation as genetic sonography, and when used as an adjunct to first- and/or second-trimester screening for Down syndrome, the detection rate is reported as high as 99% [19].

4. Genetic ultrasound in the first trimester

The genetic scan is also called nuchal scan, as NT measurement is the most important component of the first-trimester combined screen [38] which is performed between 11 weeks and 13 weeks + 6 days, when fetal crown-rump length (CRL) is between 45 and 84 mm. The scan approach is mainly transabdominal, using the transvaginal approach only in particular situations, when the visualization is poor [39]. International Society of Ultrasound in Obstetrics and Gynecology (ISUOG) guidelines recommend a minimum of technical requirements for equipment: real-time, gray-scale, two-dimensional ultrasound; transabdominal and transvaginal ultrasound transducers, adjustable acoustic power output controls with output display standards; freeze frame and zoom capabilities; electronic calipers; and capacity to print/store images [40]. An accurate dating of pregnancy according to CRL measurement is important for the screening purpose, as the values of biological markers are interpreted according the gestational age [41–43].

The most important first-trimester marker is the nuchal translucency (NT) measurement, representing the thickness of the ultrasonographic sonolucency in the posterior fetal neck, between the skin and the soft tissue overlying the cervical spine [44]. To obtain an accurate and reliable

http://dx.doi.org/10.5772/intechopen.71064

evaluation, it is necessary a sagittal view of the fetal face in the neutral position, magnification so that only the fetal head and the upper thorax are visible on the screen and the measurement of maximum thickness. Specialized training and certification are available [45, 46] (**Figure 1(A)**).

Semi-automated method of measuring NT thickness was developed, to avoid operator bias and either under- or overestimation of the measurement [47] (**Figure 2**).

Specialized software quantifies the deviation in the measured NT from the normal euploid pregnancies [47, 48]. The risk for aneuploidies, especially trisomy 21, increases exponentially with increasing NT thickness [49, 50].

The professionals should carefully explain to the patients the significance of an increased NT, as this finding has the potential to determine couples to terminate the pregnancy, worried about the possibility of an abnormal fetus [51].

4.1. Nasal bone (NB)

A common characteristic of the patients with DS is a small nose [52], and many studies have demonstrated that the absence or a hypoplastic NB in pregnancy is highly associated with

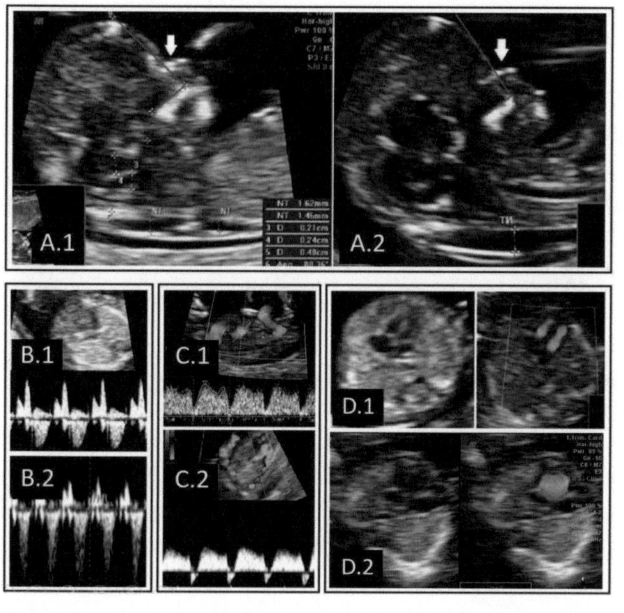

Figure 1. First-trimester ultrasound genetic markers. (A) Measurement of the cranial markers: nuchal translucency (NT), nasal bone (NB, white arrow), and fronto-maxillary facial angle (FMF, figured with red lines). (A.1) Normal values of genetic markers with small NT thickness, ossified nasal bone, and normal facial angle. (A.2) Abnormal genetic markers with increased NT thickness, absent nasal bone, and wide facial angle, of more than 90°. (B) Spectral Doppler assessment of the tricuspid flow and measurement of the fetal heart rate. (B.1) Normal tricuspid blood flow. (B.2) Regurgitation of the blood flow across the tricuspid valve. (C) Spectral Doppler assessment of the ductus venosus flow. (C.1) Normal ductal blood flow. (C.2) Abnormal ductal flow with reversed a-wave. (D) Assessment of the four-chamber view of the fetal heart in duplex mode: gray scale and color Doppler. (D.1) Normal appearance of the four-chamber view with identification of the crux cordis in gray scale and equal and separated atrioventricular flows. (D.2) Atrioventricular septal defect with common atrioventricular valve and large communication between heart cavities.

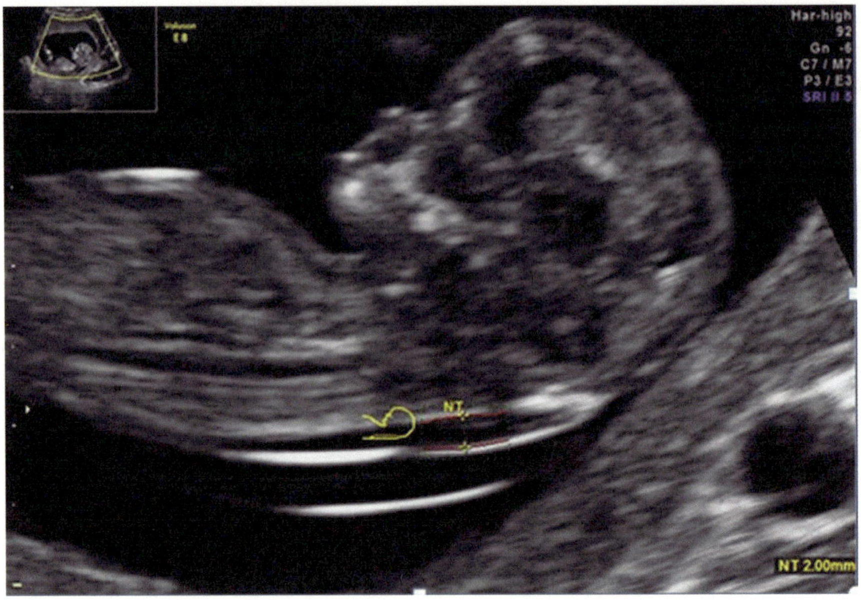

Figure 2. Semi-automated measurement of the nuchal translucency.

trisomy 21 [53, 54]. The correct evaluation of the nasal bone assumes a midsagittal view, similar to the one necessary for NT measurement. The angle of insonation should be perpendicular to the NB, which is evaluated in the so-called equal sign, with two echogenic lines (the skin of the nasal bridge and the NB underneath it) (**Figure 1(A.1)**). If the line representing the nasal bone is absent or less echogenic as the overlying skin, then the NB is noted absent or hypoplastic (**Figure 1(A.2)**) [49]. Seventy percent of trisomy 21 fetuses have absent nasal bone [55].

4.2. Doppler evaluation of the tricuspid valve: tricuspid regurgitation

Regurgitation of the blood flow across the tricuspid valve is a common marker for chromosomal defects, present in about 74% DS fetuses but also in 7% of chromosomally normal fetuses [56]. The standard evaluation is the heart apical incidence of the four-chamber view. The Doppler gate is 2–3 mm and must be placed over the tricuspid valve with a minimum angle of insonation, acceptable up to 30° (**Figure 1(B.1)**). Tricuspid regurgitation is diagnosed if reversed flow is noted more than 50% of ventricular systole and higher than 60 cm/s (**Figure 1(B.2)**) [49].

4.3. Doppler evaluation of the ductus venosus (DV)

An abnormal flow in the ductus venosus was defined as the complete cessation or a reversal forward flow of the a-wave (**Figure 1(C.2)**) but also an increased pulsatility index (PI) of the flow [57]. An accurate assessment of the ductal flow requires skilled operators since there is the possibility of interference from adjacent vessels: hepatic and umbilical veins [49]. Seventy-four percent of DS fetuses and 5% of chromosomally normal fetuses present abnormal DV flow [58].

4.4. Fronto-maxillary facial (FMF) angle

This angle is measured between the upper surface of the palate and the frontal bone (**Figure 1(A.1)**). FMF angle is significantly larger in DS fetuses (mean 88.78, range 75.4–1048) versus chromosomally normal fetuses (mean 78.18, range 66.6–89.5, P < 0.001) (**Figure 1(A.2)**) [49].

4.5. Fetal heart rate

Fetal heart rate should be measured routinely as part of DS screening. The studies have shown an increase of the fetal heart rate by 15% [59].

4.6. Fetal malformations

Another target of the first-trimester scan is to detect fetal severe malformations, which are either lethal or associated with severe handicap or aneuploidies [60, 61]. The abnormal fetuses detected early in pregnancy should be tested to exclude aneuploidy. Many major abnormalities can be diagnosed as early as the first-trimester scan [57, 62–66]. Other conditions vary in onset during gestation and do not have a consistent ultrasound appearance in the first trimester for a definitive and reliable diagnosis.

4.7. Screening in twin pregnancies

In cases of multiple gestations, the first-trimester scan should correctly diagnose the chorionicity of the pregnancy. In a monochorionic twin pregnancy, the false-positive rate of NT screening is higher than in dichorionic twins, because increased NT in at least one of the fetuses can be an early manifestation of twin-to-twin-transfusion syndrome, as well as a marker of chromosomal abnormalities [67]. It is recommended that, for the calculation of risk of trisomy 21, the NT of both twins should be measured and the average of the two should be considered [68].

An important advantage of screening by fetal NT is that when there is discordance for a chromosomal abnormality, the presence of a sonographically detectable marker helps to ensure the correct identification of the abnormal twin during selective termination.

5. Genetic ultrasound screening assessment in the second trimester

In the second trimester, the genetic ultrasound screening assessment can be used either alone or as an adjunct to maternal serum testing. The purpose of the scan is to identify fetal anomalies or chromosomal markers [69] which require invasive testing. The sonographic findings that are not generally abnormalities, but can be an indicative of fetal aneuploidy are called soft ultrasound markers. Many of them are transient. It is important to pay attention to the thickness of the nuchal fold, nasal bone appearance, or prenasal edema, but also a series of soft markers have been described: intracardiac echogenic focus, hydronephrosis, and hyperechogenic bowel were found with a higher incidence in DS fetuses than in chromosomally normal fetuses (9.6% vs. 1.5%, 17.1% vs. 5.3%, and 11.4% vs. 2.4%, respectively). The prevalence of choroid plexus cysts was not significantly different between the trisomy 21 and normal fetuses (7.5% vs. 5.0%) [70].

Nuchal fold (NF) thickness (**Figure 3(A)**) is often considered the most sensitive and most specific second-trimester marker for Down syndrome with false-positive rates as low as 1% [71]. It is measured on an axial section through the head at the level of the thalami, cavum septi pellucidi, and cerebellar hemispheres (i.e., in the same plane that is used to assess the posterior fossa structures). A NF > 5 mm has a sensitivity of 15% and a specificity of 97% in trisomy 21 detection, while a NF > 6 mm has a sensitivity of 12% and a specificity of 99% in trisomy 21 detection [71]. It is recommended that the nuchal thickness should not be measured after 20 gestational weeks.

Fetal ventriculomegaly (**Figure 3(D)**) is considered a soft marker for chromosomal abnormalities and defined as more than 10 mm across the atria of the posterior or anterior horn of lateral ventricles or alternatively, a separation of more than 3 mm of the choroid plexus from the medial wall of the lateral ventricle [72].

The nasal bone is evaluated in the standard view of fetal face profile. To define nasal bone hypoplasia (**Figure 3(E)**), many studies proposed various measurement criteria, and most cutoffs are more than 0.25 cm [73]. A hypoplastic nasal bone is seen in approximately 0.5–1.2% of normal fetuses [74].

The vast majority of cases with **choroid plexus cysts** (**Figure 3(C)**) have no associated abnormality, but still there is a soft association with aneuploidy, especially trisomy 18 and also trisomy 21. Their size and number of cysts are thought to affect the risk of aneuploidy [75]. Amniocentesis is not recommended when isolated, due to weak associations with genetic abnormalities. When the choroid plexus cysts are large (>1 cm), bilateral, multiple, or the maternal serum screening results are abnormal, and invasive testing is considered [76].

The **echogenic intracardiac focus (EIF)** represents the mineralization within the papillary muscles, usually seen at the second trimester, located in the left ventricle (**Figure 3(G)**). The association with trisomy 21 was demonstrated in up to 12% of fetuses, but biventricular EIFs are considered to be a higher risk for aneuploidy [77].

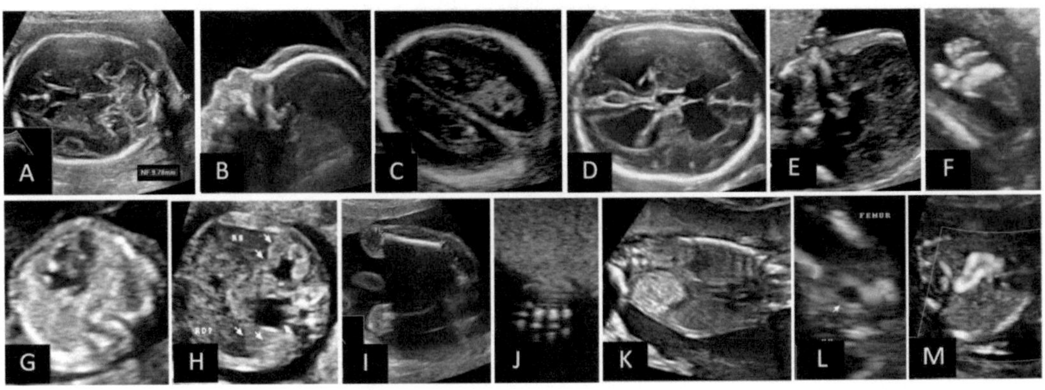

Figure 3. Second-trimester genetic markers: (A) increased thickness of the nuchal fold (NF), (B) prenasal edema, (C) bilateral choroid plexus cysts, (D) bilateral ventriculomegaly, (E) nasal bone hypoplasia, (F) gap sandals toes, (G) echogenic intracardiac focus, (H) bilateral pyelectasis/hydronephrosis, (I) measurement of femur length to detect shortening of the long bones, (J) non-visualization of the middle phalanx of the fifth digit, (K) echogenic bowel, (L) single umbilical artery, and (M) aberrant right subclavian artery.

http://dx.doi.org/10.5772/intechopen.71064

Echogenic bowel (**Figure 3(K)**) is defined if a bowel area is brighter than the bone on an image with appropriate gain settings. Trisomy 21 was diagnosed in 15% of cases, but other several associations have been reported, such as cytomegalovirus infection, cystic fibrosis, intraamniotic hemorrhage, and intrauterine growth restriction [78].

Other second-trimester soft markers for trisomy 21 include **fetal renal pyelectasis** (**Figure 3(H)**), **shortened long bones (less than third centile for gestational age) with a shortened femur or/and a shortened humerus** (**Figure 3(I)**), **single umbilical artery** (**Figure 3.(L)**), aberrant right subclavian artery (**Figure 3(M)), and gap sandals toes** (**Figure 3(F)**). When found alone, these soft markers have a weak association with DS.

As presented before, genetic sonography was used as primary screening, or as an arbitrator, to refine the initial screening result, for reassuring or when couples with positive tests did not opt for invasive testing [34, 79].

6. Cardiac anomalies (congenital heart defects, CHD)

CHD are present in the majority of the fetuses with DS [80] and represent one of the most common and lethal abnormalities present postnatally. Various heart conditions were reported

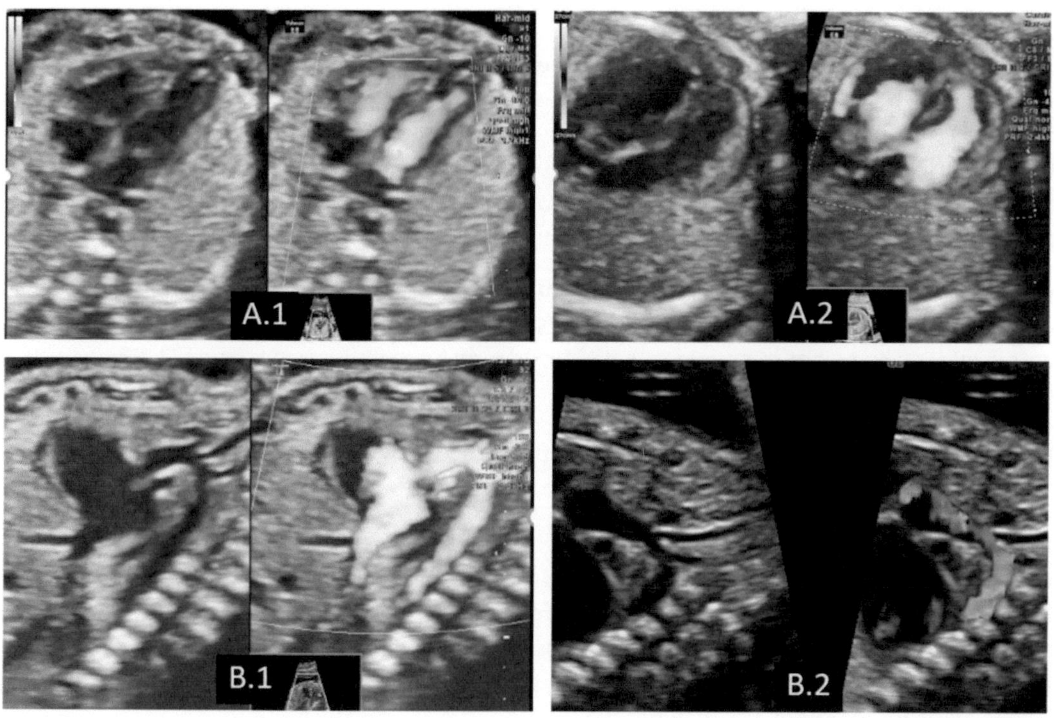

Figure 4. Congenital heart disease in DS fetuses: (A.1) normal appearance of the four-chamber view in the second trimester and atrioventricular septal defects (A.2) and (B.1) normal appearance of the aortic arch and aortic tubular stenosis (B.2).

with significant incidence [81]: ventricular, atrial, and atrioventricular septal defects (**Figure 4(A.1, A.2)**); tricuspid stenosis; outflow tract abnormalities, as Aortic coarctation **(Figure 4(B.1, B.2))**, pulmonary valve stenosis, and atresia; transposition of great vessels; common truncus; and aortic stenosis. Functional conditions, as pericardial effusion and atrioventricular regurgitation, were also noted [79].

An accurate cardiac assessment as an adjunct in the first and second trimester increases the screening power to as high as 99% [19, 34] and is the only strategy to increase the mid-trimester genetic ultrasonography detection rates over 90% [36, 79]. This may be advantageous for patients who desire the highest sensitivity for DS detection (**Figure 4**).

7. Invasive diagnostic testing

In first-trimester screening is positive for DS, chorionic villus sampling (CVS) is proposed for a definitive genetic diagnosis, by obtaining a placental tissue sample, usually transabdominally or transcervically, if the trophoblast is situated posterior. The main advantage is represented by the early diagnosis, easing the decision-making process for couples [82]. The main disadvantage is represented by the risk of spontaneous abortion that can vary from 0.6 to 4.6% [45]. Other disadvantages include the fact that is an operator-dependent procedure and that is not available in every community [83]. There is an increased risk of limb reduction defects, if the procedure is performed before 10 weeks' gestation [83].

Amniocentesis is the most common procedure for detecting genetic abnormalities before birth. A sample of the amniotic fluid is extracted usually after 15 weeks' gestation [84], because of increased abortion risk before this gestational age. The accuracy of this invasive testing is reported to be over 99.4% [85], similar to CVS. Complications are uncommon but may include vaginal spotting, amniotic fluid leakage, chorioamnionitis, failure of fetal cells to grow in culture, fetal needle injury, and fetal loss [82], in less than 1% of cases [86].

A less frequent invasive test is percutaneous umbilical blood sampling, used in the case of severe oligoamnios or for a rapid chromosome analysis (1–3 days from fetal blood vs. 10–14 days from amniocytes). The risk of miscarriage is higher than the other two procedures [82, 83].

8. Noninvasive prenatal testing (NIPT)

In the mid-1950s, the presence of fetal cells was demonstrated in the maternal circulation [87] and in 1997 also the existence of cell-free fetal DNA, which became a feasible target for a noninvasive prenatal testing [88, 89]. Fetal DNA from maternal plasma is the result of fragmented syncytiotrophoblast cells undergoing apoptosis. NIPT allows for an earlier aneuploidy detection from as early as 4 weeks' gestation [90] but is usually recommended after nine gestational weeks, in order to obtain a sufficient fetal fraction of cell-free DNA.

This Revolutionary method, with a first clinical application in determining fetal sexing, significantly reduced the gap between the performance of conventional screening and diagnostic testing [88, 91], because of the high sensitivity and specificity, especially for DS. Recently, a meta-analysis of 1963 cases of trisomy 21 and 223,932 non-trisomy 21 singleton pregnancies showed a weighted pooled detection rate of 99.7% for a false-positive rate of 0.04% [92].

NIPT is nowadays offered in conjunction with another method of screening for fetal aneuploidy rather than as a replacement. Some are concerned about losing the clinical value of the first-trimester screening, as during the last decades, this evaluation became an important pregnancy evaluation, aimed to detect the high-risk pregnancies not only for genetic abnormalities but also for structural malformations and other pregnancy severe complications. The main advantages of NIPT include the safety of the procedure, with no risk of miscarriage, the early timing, and the ease of testing, which is not "surgical," "stressful," or "painful," as invasive procedures may be. Among disadvantages, we should keep in in the costs and potential ethical issues, as the NIPT use for gender determination or the diagnosis of some conditions with variable prognosis [93, 94]. It is important to understand that NIPT is not a diagnostic test, and therefore, a positive NIPT result requires an invasive test to confirm the findings, as recommended by professional societies. Many chromosomally mosaic placentas are not detected by NIPT, and abnormal chromosome complements in maternal-derived cfDNA may be detected from apoptosis of maternal tumor cells [95].

Author details

Iliescu Dominic-Gabriel and Drăgușin Roxana-Cristina*

*Address all correspondence to: roxy_dimieru@yahoo.com

Department of Obstetrics and Gynaecology, University of Medicine and Pharmacy of Craiova, Romania

References

[1] Patterson D. Molecular genetic analysis of Down syndrome. Human Genetics. Jul 2009; **126**(1):195-214 PMID 19526251

[2] Weijerman ME, de Winter JP. Clinical practice. The care of children with Down syndrome. European Journal of Pediatrics. Dec 2010;**169**(12):1445, 52 PMC 2962780 Freely accessible. PMID 20632187

[3] American Congress of Obstetricians and Gynecologists (ACOG). (2007, May 7). ACOG's screening guidelines on chromosomal abnormalities. Retrieved 11-06-2012, from http://www.acog.org/About_ACOG/News_Room/News_Releases/2007/ACOGs_Screening_Guidelines_on_Chromosomal_Abnormalities

[4] Mansfield C, Hopfer S, Marteau TM. Termination rates after prenatal diagnosis of Down syndrome, spina bifida, anencephaly, and Turner and Klinefelter syndromes: A systematic

literature review. European Concerted Action: DADA (Decision-making After the Diagnosis of a fetal Abnormality). Prenatal Diagnosis. Sep 1999;**19**(9):808-812. PMID 10521836. DOI: 10.1002/(sici)1097-0223(199909)19:9<808::aid-pd637>3.0.co;2-b

[5] Cameron A, Macara L, Brennand J, Milton P. Screening for chromosomal abnormalities. Fetal Medicine for the MRCOG and Beyond. 2002;**1**:1-12

[6] Morris JK, Mutton DE, Alberman E. Revised estimates of the maternal age specific live birth prevalence of Down's syndrome. Journal of Medical Screening. 2002;**9**(1):2-6 PMID 11943789

[7] Zournatzi V, Daniilidis A, Karidas C, Tantanasis T, Loufopoulos A, Tzafettas J. A prospective two years study of first trimester screening for Down Syndrome. Hippokratia. 2008;**12**(1):28-32

[8] Golbus MS, Loughman WD, Epstein CJ, Halbasch G, Stephens JD, Hall BD. Prenatal genetic diagnosis in 3000 amniocenteses. The New England Journal of Medicine. 1979; **300**:157-163

[9] Merkatz IR, Nitowsky HM, Macri JN, Johnson WE. An association between low maternal serum alpha-fetoprotein and fetal chromosomal abnormalities. American Journal of Obstetrics and Gynecology. 1984;**148**:886-894

[10] Benacerraf BR, Gelman R, Frigoletto FD Jr. Sonographic identification of second-trimester fetuses with Down's syndrome. The New England Journal of Medicine. 1987; **317**:1371-1376

[11] Ginsberg N, Cadkin A, Pergament E, Verlinsky Y. Ultrasonographic detection of the second-trimester fetus with trisomy 18 and trisomy 21. American Journal of Obstetrics and Gynecology. 1990;**163**:1186-1190

[12] Cheng EY, Luthy DA, Zebelman AM, Williams MA, Lieppman RE, Hickok DE. A prospective evaluation of a second-trimester screening test for fetal Down syndrome using maternal serum alpha-fetoprotein, hCG, and unconjugated estriol. Obstetrics and Gynecology. 1993;**81**(1):72-77

[13] Watt HC, Wald NJ, George L. Maternal serum inhibin-A levels in twin pregnancies: Implications for screening for Down's syndrome. Prenatal Diagnosis. 1996;**16**:927-929

[14] Malone FD, Canick JA, Ball RH, Nyberg DA, Comstock CH, Bukowski R, Berkowitz RL, Gross SJ, Dugoff L, Craigo SD, Timor-Tritsch IE, Carr SR, Wolfe HM, Dukes K, Bianchi DW, Rudnicka AR, Hackshaw AK, Lambert-Messerlian G, Wald NJ, D'Alton ME, First- and Second-Trimester Evaluation of Risk (FASTER) Research Consortium. First-trimester or second-trimester screening, or both, for Down's syndrome. The New England Journal of Medicine. 2005;**353**:2001-2011

[15] Sheldon TA, Simpson J. Appraisal of a new scheme for prenatal screening for Down's syndrome. BMJ. 1991;**302**:1133-1136

[16] Nicolaides KH. Nuchal translucency and other first-trimester sonographic markers of chromosomal abnormalities. American Journal of Obstetrics and Gynecology. 2004; **191**:45-67

[17] Smith M, Visootsak J. Noninvasive screening tools for Down syndrome: A review. International Journal of Women's Health. 2013;**5**:125-131. DOI: 10.2147/IJWH.S31183

[18] Nicolaides KH. A model for a new pyramid of prenatal care based on the 11 to 13 weeks' assessment. Prenatal Diagnosis. 2011 Jan;**31**(1):3-6

[19] Devore GR. Genetic sonography: The historical and clinical role of fetal echocardiography. Ultrasound in Obstetrics & Gynecology. 2010 May;**35**(5):509-521

[20] CL Anderson, Brown CEL. Fetal chromosomal abnormalities: Antenatal screening and diagnosis. American Family Physician. 2009 Jan 15;**79**(2):117-123

[21] EJ Hayes & S Weiner, Universal Down syndrome testing… are we ready?, Journal Expert Review of Obstetrics & Gynecology, Volume 2, 2007 - Issue 3, Editorial, Pages 255-257

[22] ACOG Committee on Practice Bulletins. ACOG practice bulletin: Screening for fetal chromosomal abnormalities. Obstetrics and Gynecology. 2007;**109**(1):217-227

[23] Wald NJ, Rodec C, Hackshaw AK, Walters J, Chitty L, Mackinson AM. First and second trimester antenatal screening for Down's syndrome: The results of the Serum, Urine and Ultrasound Screening Study (SURUSS). Journal of Medical Screening. 2003;**10**(2):56-104

[24] National Collaborating Centre for Women's and Children's health. Antenatal Care: Routine Care for the Healthy Pregnant Woman

[25] Comstock C, Malone FD, Ball RH, et al. Is there a nuchal translucency millimeter measurement above which there is no added benefit from first trimester screening? American Journal of Obstetrics and Gynecology. 2006;**195**(3):843-847

[26] Petrovic I, Marina D, Juan CK. The role of pregnancy associated plasma protein-A (PAPP-A) in the identification of coronary artery disease activity. Acta Facultatis Medicae Naissenis. 2007;**24**(4):183-188

[27] Peterson SE, Simhan HN. First-trimester pregnancy-associated plasma protein A and subsequent abnormalities of fetal growth. American Journal of Obstetrics and Gynecology. 2008;**198**(5):43-45

[28] Bogart MH, Pandian MR, Jones OW. Abnormal maternal serum chorionic gonadotropin levels in pregnancies with fetal chromosome abnormalities. Prenatal Diagnosis. 1987;**7**:623-630

[29] Smith GC, Shah I, Crossley JA, Aitken DA, Pell JP, Nelson SM, Cameron AD, Connor MJ, Dobbie R. Pregnancy-associated plasma protein A and alpha-fetoprotein and prediction of adverse perinatal outcome. Obstetrics and Gynecology. 2006 Jan;**107**(1):161-166

[30] Shiefa S, Amargandhi M, Bhupendra J, Moulali S, Kristine T. First trimester maternal serum screening using biochemical markers papp-a and free β-hcg for down syndrome, patau syndrome and edward syndrome. Indian Journal of Clinical Biochemistry. 2013;**28**(1):3-12

[31] Wapner R, Thom E, Simpson JL, et al. First-trimester screening for trisomies 21 and 18. The New England Journal of Medicine. 2003;**349**(15):1405-1413

[32] Kagan KO, Wright D, Baker A, Sahota D, Nicolaides KH. Screening for trisomy 21 by maternal age, fetal nuchal translucency thickness, free beta-human chorionic gonadotropin and pregnancy-associated plasma protein-A. Ultrasound in Obstetrics & Gynecology. 2008;**31**:618-624

[33] Borrell A, Casals E, Fortuny A, Farre MT, Gonce A, Sanchez A, et al. First-trimester screening for trisomy 21 combining biochemistry and ultrasound at individually optimal gestational ages: An interventional study. Prenatal Diagnosis. 2004;**24**:541-545

[34] Yeo L, Vintzileos AM. The use of genetic sonography to reduce the need for amniocentesis in women at high-risk for Down syndrome. Seminars in Perinatology. 2003;**27**(2):152-159

[35] Nicolaides KH, Snijders RJ, Gosden CM, Berry C, Campbell S. Ultrasonographically detectable markers of fetal chromosomal abnormalities. Lancet. 1992;**340**(8821):704-707

[36] Vintzileos AM, Campbell WA, Rodis JF, Guzman ER, Smulian JC, Knuppel RA. The use of second-trimester genetic sonogram in guiding clinical management of patients at increased risk for fetal trisomy 21. Obstetrics and Gynecology. 1996 Jun;**87**(6):948-952

[37] Wald NJ, Watt HC, Hackshaw AK. Integrated screening for Down's syndrome based on tests performed during the first and second trimesters. The New England Journal of Medicine. 1999;**341**(7):461-467

[38] Cuckle H, Benn P, Wright D. Down syndrome screening in the first and/or second trimester: Model predicted performance using meta-analysis parameters. Seminars in Perinatology. 2005;**29**:252-257

[39] Achiron R, Tadmor O. Screening for fetal anomalies during the first trimester of pregnancy: Transvaginal versus transabdominal sonography. Ultrasound Obstet Gynecol. 1991 May 1;**1**(3):186-191

[40] Salomon LJ, Alfirevic Z, Bilardo CM, Chalouhi GE, Ghi T, Kagan KO, Lau TK, Papageorghiou AT, Raine-Fenning NJ, Stirnemann J, Suresh S, Tabor A, Timor-Tritsch IE, Toi A, Yeo G. ISUOG Practice Guidelines: Performance of first-trimester fetal ultrasound scan. Ultrasound in Obstetrics & Gynecology. 2013;**41**:102-113

[41] Crowley P. Interventions for preventing or improving the outcome of delivery at or beyond term. Cochrane Database of Systematic Reviews. 2000;**2**:CD000170

[42] Salomon LJ, Bernard M, Amarsy R, Bernard JP, Ville Y. The impact of crown–rump length measurement error on combined Down syndrome screening: A simulation study. Ultrasound in Obstetrics & Gynecology. 2009;**33**:506-511

[43] Sladkevicius P, Saltvedt S, Almström H, Kublickas M, Grunewald C, Valentin L. Ultrasound dating at 12-14 weeks of gestation. A prospective cross-validation of established dating formulae in in-vitro fertilized pregnancies. Ultrasound in Obstetrics & Gynecology. 2005;**26**:504-511

[44] Shipp TD, Benacerraf BR. Second trimester ultrasound screening for chromosomal abnormalities. Prenatal Diagnosis. 2002;**22**(4):296-307

http://dx.doi.org/10.5772/intechopen.71064

[45] Snijders RJ, Thom EA, Zachary JM, et al. First-trimester trisomy screening: Nuchal translucency measurement training and quality assurance to correct and unify technique. Ultrasound in Obstetrics & Gynecology. 2002;**19**(4):353-359

[46] Plasencia W, Dagklis T, Sotiriadis A, Borenstein M, Nicolaides KH. Frontomaxillary facial angle at 11 +0 to 13+ 6 weeks' gestation reproducibility of measurements. Ultrasound in Obstetrics & Gynecology. 2007;**29**:18-21

[47] Moratalla J, Pintoffl K, Minekawa R, et al. Semi-automated system for the measurement of nuchal translucency thickness. Ultrasound in Obstetrics & Gynecology. 2010;**36**:412-416

[48] Wright D, Kagan KO, Molina FS, Gazzoni A, Nicolaides KH. A mixture model of nuchal translucency thickness in screening for chromosomal defects. Ultrasound in Obstetrics & Gynecology. 2008;**31**:376-383

[49] Sonek J. First trimester ultrasonography in screening and detection of fetal anomalies. American Journal of Medical Genetics. Part C, Seminars in Medical Genetics. 2007;**145C**:45-61

[50] Nicolaides KH, Spencer K, Avgidou K, Faiola S, Falcon O. Multicenter study of first trimester screening for trisomy 21 in 75 821 pregnancies: Results and estimation of the potential impact of individual risk-orientated two-stage first-trimester screening. Ultrasound in Obstetrics & Gynecology. 2005;**25**:221-226

[51] Westin M, Saltvedt S, Almström H, Grunewald C, Valentin L. By how much does increased nuchal translucency increase the risk of adverse pregnancy outcome in chromosomally normal fetuses? A study of 16,260 fetuses derived from an unselected pregnant population. Ultrasound in Obstetrics & Gynecology. 2007 Feb;**29**(2):150-158

[52] Down L. Observations on an ethnic classification of idiots. Clinical Lecture Report. London Hospital; 1866;**3**:259-262

[53] Viora E, Masturzo B, Errante G, Sciarrone A, Bastonero S, Campogrande M. Ultrasound evaluation of fetal nasal bone at 11 to 14 weeks in a consecutive series of 1906 fetuses. Prenatal Diagnosis. 2003a;**23**:784-787

[54] Wong SF, Choi H, Ho LC. Nasal bone hypoplasia: Is it a common finding amongst chromosomally normal fetuses of southern Chinese women? Gynecologic and Obstetric Investigation. 2003;**56**:99-101

[55] Cicero S, Rembouskos G, Vandecruys H, Hogg M, Nicolaides KH. Likelihood ratio or Trisomy 21 in fetuses with absent nasal bone at the 11-14 weeks scan. Ultrasound in Obstetrics & Gynecology. 2004b;**23**:218-223

[56] Faiola S, Tsoi E, Huggon IC, Allan LD, Nicolaides KH. Likelihood ratio for trisomy 21 in fetuses with tricuspid regurgitation at the 11 to 13þ6 week scan. Ultrasound in Obstetrics & Gynecology. 2005;**26**:22-27

[57] Kiserud T, Eik-Nes SH, Blaas HG, Hellevik LR, Simensen B. Ductus venosus blood velocity and the umbilical circulation in the seriously growth-retarded fetus. Ultrasound in Obstetrics & Gynecology. 1994;**4**:109-114

[58] Zoppi MA, Ibba RM, Axinan C, Floris M, Manca F, Monni G. Absence of fetal nasal bone and aneuploidies at first trimester nuchal translucency screening in unselected pregnancies. Prenatal Diagnosis. 2003;**23**:496-500

[59] Hyett JA, Noble PL, Snijders RJ, Montenegro N, Nicolaides KH. Fetal heart rate in trisomy 21 and other chromosomal abnormalities at 10-14 weeks of gestation. Ultrasound in Obstetrics & Gynecology. 1996 Apr;**7**(4):239-244

[60] Souka AP, Pilalis A, Kavalakis I, Antsaklis P, Papantoniou N, Mesogitis S, Antsaklis A. Screening for major structural abnormalities at the 11- to 14-week ultrasound scan. American Journal of Obstetrics and Gynecology. 2006;**194**:393-396

[61] Snijders RJM, Farrias M, von Kaisenberg C, Nicolaides KH. 1996. Fetal abnormalities. In: Snijders RJM, Nicolaides KH, editors. Ultrasound Markers for Fetal Chromosomal Defects. Carnforth, UK: Parthenon Publishing. pp. 1-62

[62] Johnson SP, Sebire NJ, Snijders RJM, Tunkel S, Nicolaides KH. Ultrasound screening for anencephaly at 10-14 weeks of gestation. Ultrasound in Obstetrics & Gynecology. 1997;**9**:14-16

[63] Sepulveda W, Sebire NJ, Souka A, Snijders RJM, Nicolaides KH. Diagnosis of Meckel-Gruber syndrome at eleven to fourteen weeks' gestation. American Journal of Obstetrics and Gynecology. 1997;**176**:316-319

[64] Lin Y, Chang F, Liu C. Antenatal detection of hydranencephaly at 12 weeks menstrual age. Journal of Clinical Ultrasound. 1992;**20**:62-64

[65] Tudorache S, Iliescu DG, Turcu A, Florea M, Dragusin R, Novac L, Nicolae C, Cernea D. First trimester anomaly scan-the last redoubt won: Open spina bifida. Donald School Journal of Ultrasound in Obstetrics and Gynecology. 2015;**9**(1):80-90

[66] Guzman ER. Early prenatal diagnosis of gastroschisis with transvaginal sonography. American Journal of Obstetrics and Gynecology. 1990;**162**:1253-1254

[67] Kagan KO, Gazzoni A, Sepulveda-Gonzalez G, Sotiriadis A, Nicolaides KH. Discordance in nuchal translucency thickness in the prediction of severe twin-to-twin transfusion syndrome. Ultrasound in Obstetrics & Gynecology. 2007;**29**:527-532

[68] Vandecruys H, Faiola S, Auer M, Sebire N, Nicolaides KH. Screening for trisomy 21 in monochorionic twins by measurement of fetal nuchal translucency thickness. Ultrasound in Obstetrics & Gynecology. 2005;**25**:551-553

[69] Salomon LJ, Alfirevic Z, Berghella V, Bilardo C, Hernandez-Andrade E, Johnsen SL, Kalache K, Leung K-Y, Malinger G, Munoz H, Prefumo F, Toi A, Lee W, on behalf of the ISUOG Clinical Standards Committee. Practice guidelines for performance of the routine mid-trimester fetal ultrasound scan. Ultrasound in Obstetrics & Gynecology. 2011;**37**:116-126

[70] Dagklis T, Plasencia W, Maiz N, Duarte L, Nicolaides KH. Choroid plexus cyst, intracardiac echogenic focus, hyperechogenic bowel and hydronephrosis in screening for trisomy 21 at 11 + 0 to 13 + 6 weeks. Ultrasound in Obstetrics & Gynecology. 2008 Feb;**31**(2):132-135

[71] Locatelli A, Piccoli MG, Vergani P, et al. Critical appraisal of the use of nuchal fold thickness measurements for the prediction of Down syndrome. American Journal of Obstetrics and Gynecology. 2000;**182**(1 Pt 1):192-197

[72] Wyldes M, Watkinson M. Isolated mild fetal ventriculomegaly. Archives of Disease in Childhood. Fetal and Neonatal Edition. 2004;**89**(1):F9-F13

[73] Cicero S, Sonek JD, Mckenna DS, et al. Nasal bone hypoplasia in trisomy 21 at 15-22 weeks' gestation. Ultrasound in Obstetrics & Gynecology. 2003;**21**(1):15-18. DOI: 10.1002/uog.19

[74] Kumar S. Handbook of Fetal Medicine. Cambridge University Press; 2010 ISBN: 0521675367

[75] Norton KI, Rai B, Desai H, et al. Prevalence of choroid plexus cysts in term and near-term infants with congenital heart disease. AJR. American Journal of Roentgenology. 2011;**196**(3):W326-W329

[76] Lopez JA, Reich D. Choroid plexus cysts. Journal of American Board of Family Medicine. 2006;**19**(4):422-425

[77] Anderson N, Jyoti R. Relationship of isolated fetal intracardiac echogenic focus to trisomy 21 at the mid-trimester sonogram in women younger than 35 years. Ultrasound in Obstetrics & Gynecology: The Official Journal of the International Society of Ultrasound in Obstetrics and Gynecology. 2003;**21**(4):354-358

[78] Bahado-Singh R, Morotti R, Copel JA, et al. Hyperechoic fetal bowel: The perinatal consequences. Prenatal Diagnosis. 1995;**14**(10):981-987

[79] DeVore GR. Trisomy 21: 91% detection rate using second trimester ultrasound markers. Ultrasound in Obstetrics & Gynecology. 2010;**16**:133-141

[80] Paladini D, Tartaglione A, Agangi A, Teodoro A, Forleo F, Borghese A, Martinelli P. The association between congenital heart disease and Down syndrome in prenatal life. Ultrasound in Obstetrics & Gynecology. 2000;**15**:104-108

[81] Cleves MA, Hobbs CA, Cleves PA, Tilford JM, Bird TM, Robbins JM. Congenital defects among liveborn infants with Down syndrome. Birth Defects Research. Part A, Clinical and Molecular Teratology. 2007 Sep;**79**(9):657-663

[82] Cunningham FG, Leveno KL, Bloom SL, Hauth JC, Gilstrap LC III, Wenstrom KD. Williams Obstetrics. 22nd ed. New York, NY: McGraw-Hill; 2005. p. 328-330

[83] Jenkins TM, Wapner RJ. Prenatal diagnosis of congenital disorders. In: Creasy RK, Resnik R, editors. Maternal-Fetal Medicine: Principles and Practice. 5th ed. W. B. Saunders: Philadelphia, PA; 2004. p. 263-269

[84] Alfirevic Z, Sundberg K, Brigham S. Amniocentesis and chorionic villus sampling for prenatal diagnosis. Cochrane Database of Systematic Reviews. 2003;**3**:CD003252

[85] Rhoads GG, Jackson LG, Schlesselman SE, et al. The safety and efficacy of chorionic villus sampling for early prenatal diagnosis of cytogenetic abnormalities. The New England Journal of Medicine. 1989;**320**(10):609-617

[86] Tabor A, Philip J, Madsen M, Bang J, Obel EB, Nørgaard-Pedersen B. Randomised controlled trial of genetic amniocentesis in 4606 low-risk women. Lancet. 1986; **1**(8493):1287-1293

[87] Wright CF, Burton H. The use of cell-free fetal nucleic acids in maternal blood for non-invasive prenatal diagnosis. Human Reproduction Update. 2009;**15**:139-151

[88] Lo Y, Corbetta N, Chamberlain PF, et al. Presence of fetal DNA in maternal plasma and serum. Lancet. 1997;**350**:485-487

[89] Benn P. Non-invasive prenatal testing using cell free DNA in maternal plasma: Recent developments and future prospects. Journal of Clinical Medicine. 2014;**3**(2):537-565

[90] Webb A, Madgett T, Miran T, Sillence K, Kaushik N, Kiernan M, Avent N. Non invasive prenatal diagnosis of aneuploidy: Next generation sequencing or fetal DNA enrichment? Balkan Journal of Medical Genetics: BJMG. 2012 Dec;**15**(Suppl):17-26

[91] Tounta G, Kolialexi A, Papantoniou N, Tsangaris GT, Kanavakis E, Mavrou A. Non-invasive prenatal diagnosis using cell-free fetal nucleic acids in maternal plasma: Progress overview beyond predictive and personalized diagnosis. The EPMA Journal. 2011;**2**(2):163-171

[92] Gil MM, Accurti V, Santacruz B, Plana MN, Nicolaides KH. Analysis of cell-free DNA in maternal blood in screening for aneuploidies: Updated meta-analysis. Ultrasound in Obstetrics & Gynecology. 2017;**50**:302-314

[93] Suskin E, Hercher L, Aaron KE, Bajaj K. The integration of noninvasive prenatal screening into the existing prenatal paradigm: A survey of current genetic counseling practice. Journal of Genetic Counseling. 2016 Oct;**25**(5):1032-1043

[94] Lewis C, Hill M, Skirton H, Chitty LS. Non-invasive prenatal diagnosis for fetal sex determination: Benefits and disadvantages from the service users' perspective. European Journal of Human Genetics. 2012;**20**(11):1127-1133

[95] Lebo RV, Novak RW, Wolfe K, Michelson M, Robinson H, Mancuso MS. Discordant circulating fetal DNA and subsequent cytogenetics reveal false negative, placental mosaic, and fetal mosaic cfDNA genotypes. Journal of Translational Medicine. 2015;**13**:260

Section 4

Diseases Associated with Down Syndrome

Chapter 6

Congenital Heart Disease in Down Syndrome

Margaret Louise Morrison and Colin J. McMahon

Additional information is available at the end of the chapter

http://dx.doi.org/10.5772/intechopen.71060

Abstract

Down syndrome remains the most common chromosomal abnormality in live-born infants in the world today. The association between Down syndrome and congenital heart disease (CHD) is well known, and it is widely recognized that CHD contributes significantly to the morbidity of children with Down syndrome. The reported incidence of CHD in Down syndrome patients is between 40 and 60%. The most commonly described defect is complete atrioventricular septal defect (AVSD), which comprises 30–40% of all cardiac defects. Complex genetic factors are involved. Routine cardiac screening of all newborn babies with Down syndrome is recommended. Expert groups suggest that the cardiac status of all children with Down syndrome should be established by 6 weeks of age to permit appropriate and timely treatment avoiding the establishment of irreversible pulmonary vascular disease that would make corrective surgery impossible.

Keywords: Down syndrome, congenital heart disease, screening, AVSD, pulmonary hypertension

1. Introduction

Down syndrome remains the most common chromosomal abnormality in live-born infants in the world today [1]. The association between Down syndrome and congenital heart disease (CHD) is well known. It is widely recognized that CHD contributes significantly to the morbidity and mortality of children with Down syndrome. Despite this there continues to be reports of children with Down syndrome who present with serious CHD too late for the best chance of a good cardiac outcome [2]. Early recognition of lesions is pivotal to obtain the best possible outcome, and education is still needed. In this chapter, we discuss the incidence and main types of CHD occurring in the setting of Down syndrome. We focus mainly on atrioventricular septal defect (AVSD), which accounts for 30–40% of all cardiac defects in Down syndrome patients. We review genetic consideration and also discuss the principles of surveillance for cardiac disease in this population.

2. Prevalence and genetics

Prevalence of Down syndrome is estimated to be around 1–2 per 1000 live births [1]. The reported incidence of CHD in Down syndrome patients is between 40 and 60% [1–3]. The most commonly described defect is complete AVSD which comprises 30–40% of all cardiac defects. The types of CHD described in Down syndrome do seem to follow a fixed pattern; there are high numbers of septal defects in general; tetralogy of Fallot is described, but there are lower rates of other conotruncal defects like transposition or conditions such as coarctation [4]. Prevalence of individual lesions is given later in **Table 1**.

Obviously the triplication of chromosome 21 suggests that genes located in this area are likely to play an important role in the development of CHD. However the fact that Down syndrome is not invariably accompanied by CHD implies that more complex genetic factors are involved. No single gene candidate has been identified yet [1]. Recent research implicates Hsa21-encoded genes in the development of CHD [5]. Genes for several matrix-related proteins COL-α1 and COL-α2 and Down syndrome cell adhesion molecule (DSCM) are located in chromosome 21. Overexpression of these genes for collagen matrix-related proteins has been associated with development of AVSD [4]. However not all AVSDs are associated with trisomy 21. Other genes not located on chromosome 21 and environmental factors may play a role [1, 5].

Mutations in the cell adhesion molecule cysteine-rich epidermal growth factor-like domain (CRELD) 1 on chromosome 3 have also been implicated in the genetics of CHD in Down syndrome and correspond to one of the specific genetic loci identified for AVSD [6]. This molecule is thought to be essential to the process of cellular adhesion and formation of the endocardial cushions. Overexpression of the junction adhesion molecule (JAM) 2 has also been shown to potentiate CHD in mice that already have CRELD1 mutation [7]. Undoubtedly the genetic influence of chromosome 21 on CHD is complex and yet to be fully understood.

There is evidence to suggest that sex and ethnic differences do exist in the incidence of CHD in Down syndrome, particularly among those with AVSD. There is a predominance of female infants

	Percentage of Down syndrome patients affected by study			
	Tubman et al. [3]	**Frid et al. [17]**	**Freeman et al. [8]**	**Stoll et al. [18]**
AVSD	38%	47%	39%	30%
VSD	15%	33%	43%	22%
ASD	21%	8%	42%	25%
Tetralogy of Fallot	—	2%	6%	3%
Coarctation	—	1%	—	5%
TGA	—	—	—	—
Patent ductus	18%	9%	—	5%

Table 1. Percentage of patients with Down syndrome affected by congenital heart disease by defect.

http://dx.doi.org/10.5772/intechopen.71060

affected by AVSD and VSD [8]. Black infants with Down syndrome appear to have around twice the risk of AVSD as white infants, whereas Hispanic infants have a much smaller risk than white infants [8]. The type of lesion is thought to vary according to geographical area. For example, in Brazil the most frequently described defect is an atrial septal defect (ASD) [9, 10]. In Asia the most common lesion is a ventricular septal defect (VSD) [11]. A group in Sweden reports AVSD as the most frequent lesion like other Western European countries and the USA. Interestingly they also note a decreasing frequency of complex CHD in Down syndrome; such a trend could be explained by selective termination of fetuses with Down syndrome in some areas [12].

3. Surveillance and screening

The American Academy of Pediatrics recommends routine cardiac screening of all newborn babies with Down syndrome [13]. This statement is echoed by the Down Syndrome Medical Interest group (DSMIG UK). They recommend that the cardiac status of all children with Down syndrome should be established by 6 weeks of age [2]. Age at evaluation is an important factor for reduction in morbidity and mortality rates. Failure to recognize cardiac defects early in life can have serious consequences including establishment of irreversible pulmonary vascular disease that makes corrective surgery impossible [3]. The fact that children still occasionally present to pediatric cardiology clinics in this fashion indicates that the importance of early detection is not fully acknowledged, even in the present era [9, 14]. Neonatal and infant mortality in patients with Down syndrome remains higher than in the general population, primarily due to CHD [1].

Clinical examination alone remains insufficient to reliably diagnose CHD in Down syndrome with only around 40% of newborns having a cardiovascular abnormality detected based solely on clinical findings [3, 15]. An ECG is likely to be abnormal, particularly in the setting of AVSD, and an abnormal ECG has been shown to have a high positive predictive value for congenital heart disease [3]. Taken together clinical examination and ECG are more powerful than either individually [3].

Echocardiography is undoubtedly the most effective single diagnostic test however even it is not 100% effective in identifying lesions in the neonatal period. Authors acknowledge that echocardiography should only be carried out by pediatric cardiologists or experienced pediatricians with special interest in cardiology that have access to the necessary equipment and technical skills [3, 15]. There should be a low threshold for repeating the investigation if symptoms or signs of cardiac disease present at any age, even with a history of previously normal echocardiogram [2]. Diagnosis of purely physiological shunts such a PFO or PDA may cause unnecessary worry for some parents.

The DSMIG suggest that all babies with a diagnosis of Down syndrome should have a thorough clinical examination and ECG performed shortly after diagnosis and that the urgency of their assessment by a pediatric cardiologist should be determined on the basis of these investigations, such that those with abnormal signs or abnormal ECG be seen within 2 weeks for echocardiogram and those felt to be at lower risk based on the initial tests be seen within 6 weeks from birth [2].

4. Common cardiac defects occurring in Down syndrome

The major types of congenital heart defect occurring in Down syndrome are listed in **Table 1**. As noted earlier the most common defect is AVSD, which can affect up to 40% of patients [1]. Conversely around 80% of all AVSDs occur in children with Down syndrome [16]. We describe the morphology and pathophysiology of some of the major types of CHD associated with Down syndrome.

AVSD, atrioventricular septal defect; VSD, ventricular septal defect; ASD, atrial septal defect; TGA, transposition of the great arteries.

4.1. Atrioventricular septal defect (AVSD)

The term AVSD covers a broad spectrum of CHD characterized by a common atrioventricular junction with coexisting deficiency in the atrioventricular septum. AVSD comprises around 7% of all CHD and is also referred to as an endocardial cushion defect [19].

The common atrioventricular junction is usually ovoid with unwedging of the left ventricular outflow tract from the usual position between mitral and tricuspid valves. Instead of separate inlet valves, the AV junction is guarded by a common valve, which often is comprised of five leaflets, two of which are bridging leaflets across the crest of the interventricular septum (**Figure 1**). These are termed superior and inferior bridging leaflets, respectively. There is also a left lateral (mural) leaflet, right anterosuperior leaflet, and a right inferior leaflet [16, 19].

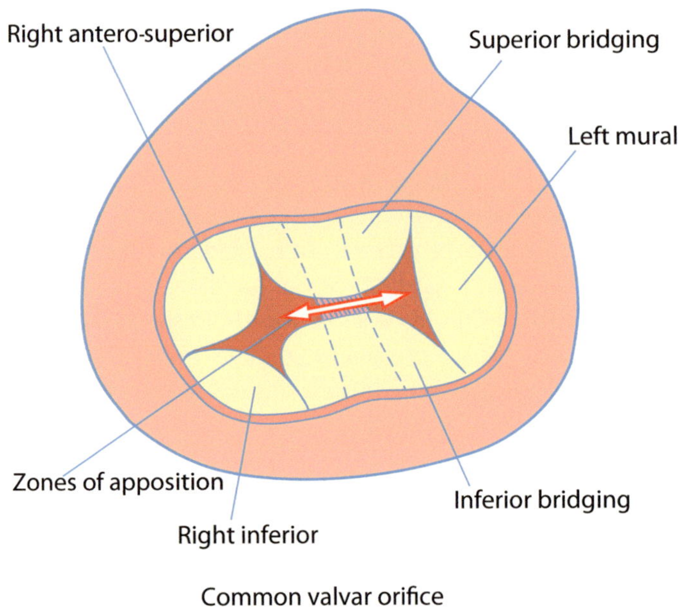

Figure 1. The arrangement of the common atrioventricular valve leaflets in complete AVSD.

The Rastelli classification from 1966 divides complete AVSD into three subgroups on the basis of the anatomy of the superior bridging leaflet and its chordal attachments (**Figure 2**). In Rastelli type A, the superior bridging leaflet is divided at the level of the ventricular septum; in Rastelli type B, the division of the superior bridging leaflet occurs to a right ventricular papillary muscle; and in Rastelli type C, the superior bridging leaflet is undivided or free floating. Rastelli type C is the most common arrangement found in Down syndrome [20].

In complete AVSD, shunting occurs at both atrial and ventricular levels; however, attachment of the bridging leaflets to the crest of ventricular septum results in an exclusively atrial shunt through a primum ASD, also called a partial AVSD (see later), whereas attachment of the bridging leaflet to the atrial septum results in exclusively ventricular shunting (**Figure 3**).

Other congenital heart defects commonly associated with AVSD include left ventricular outflow tract obstruction especially in the setting of a Rastelli type A superior bridging leaflet as there is extreme unwedging of the aorta from its usual position and consequent elongation of the outflow tract. Ventricular hypoplasia and atrial isomerism are also described although infrequently with Down syndrome. Tetralogy of Fallot is the most commonly observed association and is seen in up to 6.7% cases of AVSD [20]. There is a high incidence of associated other extra cardiac abnormalities. One study of 87 patients with Tetralogy and AVSD reported that 67% of these patients had Down syndrome [21].

Clinical presentation relates to the morphology of the AVSD and any associated defects. If the ventricular component is large, left to right shunting occurs after the first few weeks of life as the pulmonary vascular resistance falls, and the infant will develop signs of congestive heart failure.

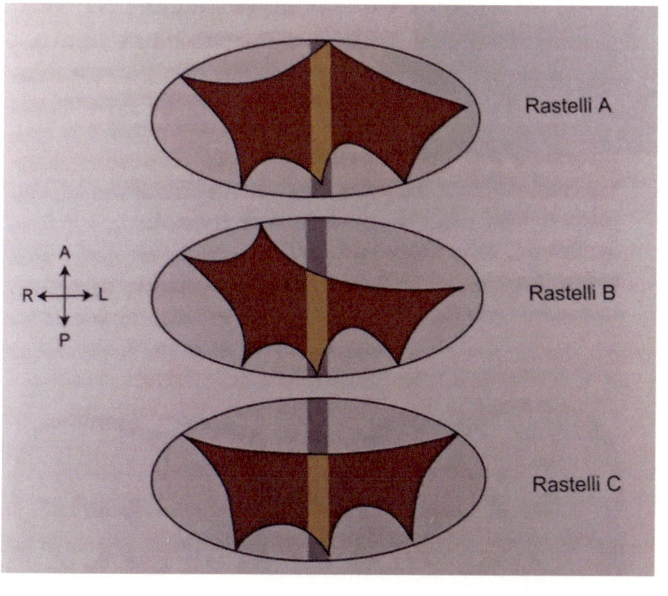

Figure 2. Rastelli classification. Type a (top): The superior bridging leaflet is divided at the ventricular septum. Type B (middle): The division occurs to a right ventricular papillary muscle. Type C (bottom): The superior bridging leaflet is undivided.

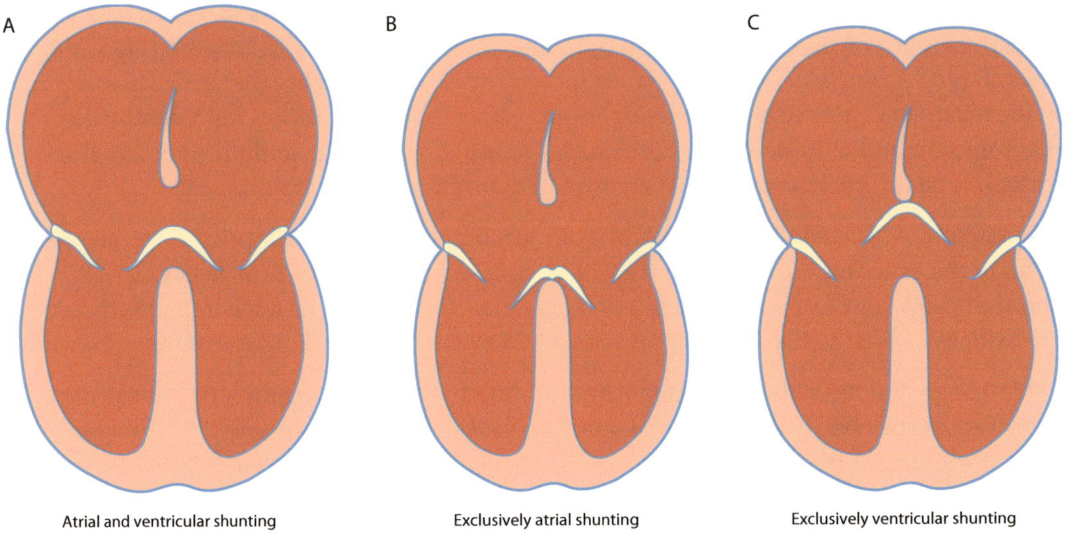

Figure 3. Resultant shunting in complete AVSD depends on the arrangement of the bridging leaflets with the atrial and ventricular septum. (A) atrial and ventricular shunting, (B) exclusively atrial shunting, (C) exclusively ventricular shunting.

If there is associated significant AV valve regurgitation, ventricular imbalance or coarctation signs of cardiac failure will occur much earlier [16, 20]. There is a small subgroup of patients with complete AVSD who do not develop signs of cardiac failure despite a significant ventricular component. In these individuals there is persistent elevation of pulmonary vascular resistance [20].

In the present era, medical treatment is aimed at optimizing the patient's condition to get to corrective surgery. This includes maximizing fluids and calorie intake, often with supplemental nasogastric tube feeding to promote good nutrition. Symptomatic management of congestive heart failure is with diuretics and ACE inhibitor therapy. The aim of surgery is to completely close the septal defects and repair the AV valve. Today surgery is offered to all Down syndrome patients with CHD although this was not always the case. Surgical results are good, and there is believed to be no extra risk from the concomitant presence of Down syndrome [22, 23]. Surgical repair is aimed in the first few months of life and certainly before 6 months old as irreversible pulmonary vascular disease is more likely to develop quickly in patients with Down syndrome and AVSD. Surgery is usually successful with low operative mortality. The most recent statistics from National Institute for Cardiovascular Outcomes Research (NICOR) suggest that survival following complete AVSD repair is 99.5% at 30 days post-op and 91.9% at 1 year [24]. Without corrective surgery many patients with complete AVSD will die in infancy, with only 4% surviving beyond 5 years old [25]. Those who survive will develop pulmonary vascular disease and eventual reversal of the systemic to pulmonary shunt with accompanying cyanosis or Eisenmenger's syndrome.

Postoperative complications following surgical repair of complete AVSD are listed in **Table 2**. Those seen most commonly are left ventricular outflow tract obstruction and left AV valve regurgitation. Left AV valve regurgitation forms the most common reason for reoperation in

• Left atrioventricular valve regurgitation
• Left ventricular outflow tract obstruction
• Late-onset complete heart block
• Pulmonary vascular disease
• Atrial or ventricular rhythm problems
• Left atrioventricular valve stenosis
• Right atrioventricular valve stenosis or regurgitation
• Residual ventricular septal defect
• Aortic incompetence

Table 2. Long-term complications following repair of complete AVSD [16, 19].

most surgical series [26]. Interestingly, the morphology of the AV valve most associated with Down syndrome, Rastelli type C, may actually be more favorable for surgical repair as there is often extensive bridging of both superior and inferior bridging leaflets resulting in less left AV valve regurgitation. Surgical series demonstrate that patients with Down syndrome experience greater freedom from reoperation for left AV valve regurgitation than those without Down syndrome [27].

4.2. Primum atrial septal defect/partial AVSD

In an isolated primum ASD or partial AVSD, the AV junction is a common structure; however, there are separate right and left AV valve orifices as a band of valve tissue joins the superior and inferior bridging leaflets. The AV valves appear at the same level, and there may be regurgitation through the zone of opposition or "cleft" in the left AV valve (**Figure 4**). Timing of surgery in this case is less crucial especially if there is minimal AV valve regurgitation. Repair is often carried out in late infancy or early childhood. Isolated primum ASD unrepaired carries 50% mortality before the age of 20 years [16]. Surgical results are good, and 30-day and 1-year survival are 98.8 and 98.7%, respectively [24]. Long-term complications are similar to those described following AVSD repair with the most common reason for reoperation being left AV valve regurgitation followed by left ventricular outflow tract obstruction [26].

4.3. Tetralogy of Fallot

Tetralogy of Fallot is a conotruncal defect caused by the anterior and cephalad deviation of the infundibular septum, which leads to the development of the four characteristic components: ventricular septal defect, overriding aorta, right ventricular outflow tract obstruction, and right ventricular hypertrophy (**Figure 5**). Tetralogy of Fallot occurs in around 6% of patients with Down syndrome and is the most common cyanotic heart defect to present in this patient group. Conversely around 8% of patients with Tetralogy of Fallot have Down syndrome, although this is slightly higher in fetal series [28].

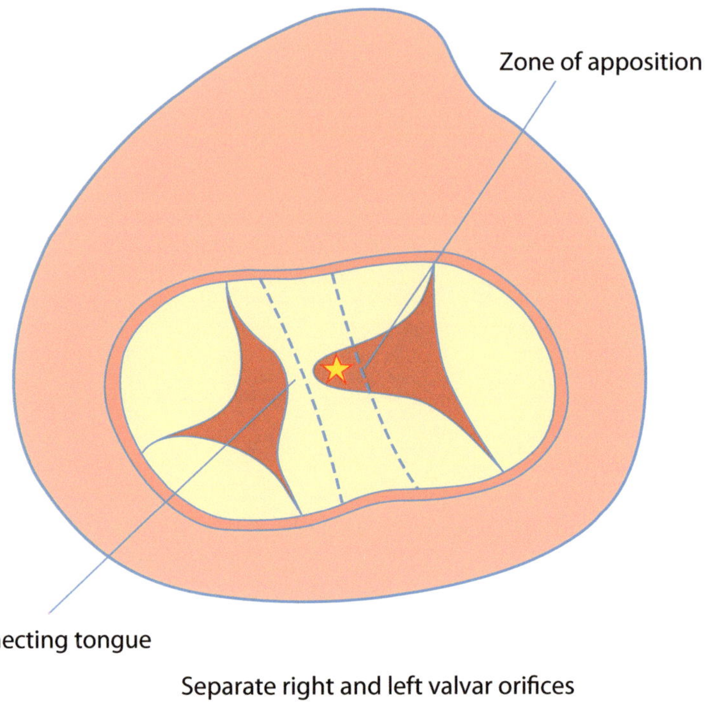

Figure 4. Arrangement of the common atrioventricular valve leaflets in primum ASD.

Clinical presentation of tetralogy of Fallot depends very much on the degree of outflow tract obstruction present. Patients may present with profound central cyanosis in the neonatal period if the obstruction is severe and may actually be duct dependent, i.e., there is insufficient pulmonary blood flow once the ductus arteriosus closes. These patients require palliation with a Blalock-Taussig shunt or ductal stent to secure pulmonary blood flow and permit growth for corrective surgery. If there is little outflow tract obstruction, the patient may exhibit signs and symptoms of congestive cardiac failure as there will be a large left to right shunt through the VSD; in this case there will be little or no cyanosis.

Most commonly, patients fall somewhere in between and have a degree of outflow tract obstruction often presenting with an ejection systolic murmur and some cyanosis [28]. The degree of cyanosis is often variable, and patients may have cyanotic spells, which result from an acute increase in right to left shunting due to spasm of the muscular infundibular region. Patients with cyanosis or frequent spells that cannot be managed with beta blocker therapy may require a RVOT stent. Corrective surgery is performed at around 6–8 months of age. Outcomes are good, and survival following tetralogy repair is 99.7% at 30 days and 97.8% at 1 year [24]. Common long-term complications are listed in **Table 3**.

The relief of right ventricular outflow tract obstruction during tetralogy of Fallot repair results in chronic pulmonary regurgitation, which subsequently leads to right ventricular dilatation

http://dx.doi.org/10.5772/intechopen.71060

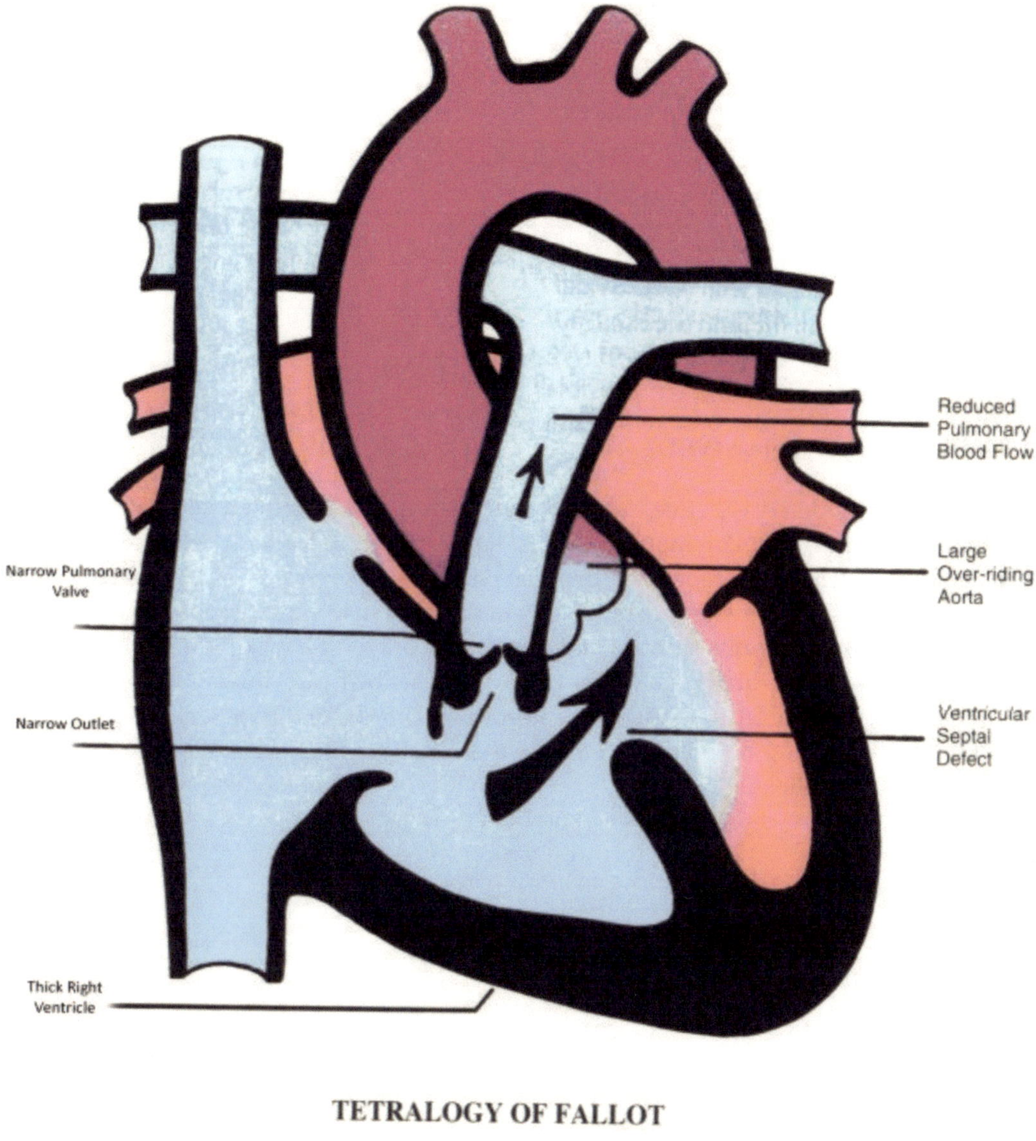

Figure 5. Diagrammatic representation of tetralogy of Fallot.

necessitating interventions. The most frequent reason for reoperation in this patient group is to replace the pulmonary valve either surgically or percutaneously [28, 29]. There is evidence to suggest that patients with Down syndrome who have undergone tetralogy of Fallot repair come to pulmonary valve replacement more frequently than patients without Down syndrome. This is felt to be due to the presence of pulmonary arterial hypertension, also common in Down syndrome, which contributes to more severe pulmonary regurgitation and earlier RV dilatation [30].

• Pulmonary regurgitation
• Right ventricular dilatation and dysfunction
• Residual right ventricular outflow tract obstruction
• Branch pulmonary stenosis
• Rhythm problems
• Aortic incompetence
• Aortic root dilatation

Table 3. Long-term complications following tetralogy of Fallot repair [29].

4.4. Ventricular septal defect (VSD)

A ventricular septal defect is defined as a hole between the right and left ventricles. In most series it is the second most common form of CHD described in Down syndrome (**Table 1**). VSDs are generally classified depending on what portion of the ventricular septum they span, illustrated in **Figure 6**. In Down syndrome VSDs often occur in the inlet septum [31]. In a large series of patients with Down syndrome, inlet VSD was one of the most frequently reported subtypes. Muscular and subarterial VSDs were not described [32]. Inlet VSD is associated with abnormalities of the left AV valve with straddling chordal and papillary muscle attachments [31]. In the setting of Down syndrome, these defects likely form part of the AVSD complex described earlier [32].

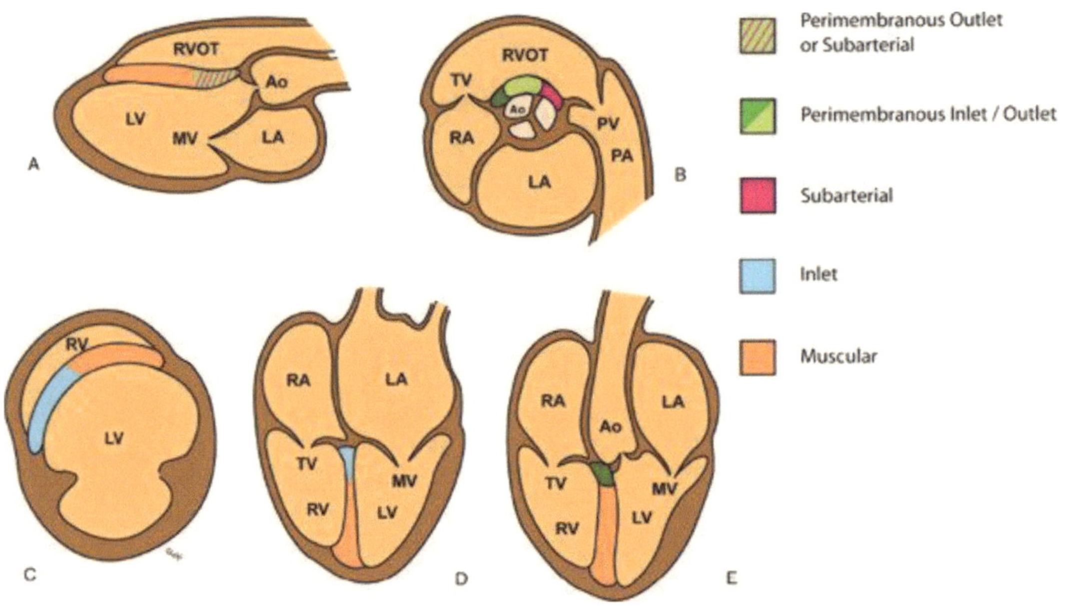

Figure 6. Diagrammatic representation of possible VSD locations on standard echo views. (A) long axis view, (B) short axis view at aortic valve level, (C) short axis view through ventricles, (D) four chamber view, (E) left ventricular outflow tract view.

Similarly to AVSD, a VSD results in a left to right shunt with extra pulmonary blood flow, the magnitude of which depends on both the size of the defect and the patient's pulmonary vascular resistance. Hemodynamically significant defects are repaired before 6 months of age. Like AVSD uncorrected lesions will lead to the development of pulmonary vascular disease and Eisenmenger's syndrome [31].

4.5. Other lesions

From late adolescence there is evidence of an increased incidence of asymptomatic mitral valve prolapse (MVP) and aortic incompetence in children with Down syndrome. These are often asymptomatic; however, the MVP in particular can progress to symptomatic mitral regurgitation, and it is recommended that auscultation continues to be part of surveillance for individuals with Down syndrome in adult life [2].

5. Pulmonary hypertension in Down syndrome

Patients with Down syndrome are considered to be at higher risk of pulmonary arterial hypertension both with and without CHD. This is likely to be multifactorial, but the high incidence of CHD and airway problems undoubtedly plays a pivotal role in its development [33]. Down syndrome patients have a high incidence of gastroesophageal reflux with micro-aspiration, recurrent respiratory infections, and sleep apnea. They may experience chronic hypoxia from upper airway obstruction in the form of tracheobronchomalacia, stenosis, or subglottic compromise [33]. There is a high prevalence of persistent pulmonary hypertension of the newborn in infants with Down syndrome, and as discussed earlier, there is a small subset of Down syndrome CHD patients who continue to have elevated pulmonary vascular resistance beyond the newborn period [16].

In the setting of a significant left to right shunt, intrinsic lung abnormalities such as abnormal pulmonary arterioles, a smaller number of alveoli, and impaired endothelial function contribute to the development of pulmonary arterial hypertension in association with CHD [34]. As observed earlier, timely corrective surgery will prevent irreversible lung damage and development of Eisenmenger's syndrome. Despite this move to early surgery, there remain a significant number of Down syndrome patients with Eisenmenger's syndrome among the adult congenital heart disease population. Some studies estimate that as many as 50% of the total population of Eisenmenger's patients have Down syndrome; there is also evidence to suggest that this group receives significantly less therapy and is often under-managed [35].

6. Conclusions

Congenital heart disease is one of the most frequent associations with Down syndrome and remains a major cause of morbidity and mortality among patients. Over half of Down syndrome patients have CHD the most common form being complete AVSD. Ethnic and geographical variations among lesions have been described. Early recognition of lesions is paramount to permit appropriate and timely treatment. To this end, cardiac screening should be undertaken in all newborn infants with Down syndrome.

Author details

Margaret Louise Morrison and Colin J. McMahon*

*Address all correspondence to: cmcmahon992004@yahoo.com

Department of Paediatric Cardiology, Our Lady's Hospital for Sick Children, Crumlin, Dublin, Ireland

References

[1] Vis JC, MGJ D, Winter MM, et al. Down syndrome: A cardiovascular perspective. Journal of Intellectual Disability Research. 2009;**53**:419-425

[2] DSMIG UK. Guidelines for Sssential Medical Surveillance for People with Down Syndrome. 2007. Available form: http://dsmig.org.uk/library/articles/guideline-cardiac-5.pdf. [Accessed: August 31, 2017]

[3] Tubman TRJ, Shields MD, Craig BG, et al. Congenital heart disease in Down syndrome: Two year prospective early screening study. British Medical Journal. 1991;**302**:1425-1427

[4] Colvin KL, Yeager ME. What people with Down syndrome can teach us about cardiopulmonary disease. European Respiratory Review. 2017;**26**:160098

[5] Asim A, Kumar A, Muthuswamy S, et al. Down syndrome: An insight of the disease. Journal of Biomedical Science. 2015;**22**:41

[6] Priestly MD, Water J, Maliszewska C, et al. Detailed mapping of a congenital heart disease gene in chromosome 3p25. Journal of Medical Genetics. 2000;**37**:581-587

[7] Li H, Edie S, Klinedinst D, et al. Penetrance of congenital heart disease in a mouse model of Down syndrome depends on a trisomic potentiator of a disomic modifier. Genetics. 2016;**203**:763-770

[8] Freeman SB, Bean LH, Allen EG, et al. Ethnicity, sex and the incidence of congenital heart defects: A report from the national Down syndrome project. Genetics in Medicine. 2008;**10**:173-180

[9] Mourato FA, Villachan LRR, de Silva Mattos S. Prevalence and profile of congenital heart disease and pulmonary hypertension in Down syndrome in a pediatric cardiology service. The Revista Paulista de Pediatria 2014;**32**:159-163

http://dx.doi.org/10.5772/intechopen.71060

[10] Bermudez BEBV, Medeiros SL, Bermudez MB, et al. Down syndrome: Prevalence and distribution of congenital heart disease in Brazil. São Paulo Medical Journal. 2015;**133**:621-624

[11] Jacobs EG, Leung MP, Karlberg J. Distribution of symptomatic congenital heart disease in Hong Kong. Pediatric Cardiology. 2000;**21**:148-157

[12] Bergstrom S, Carr H, Ptereson G, et al. Trends in congenital heart defects in infants with Down syndrome. Pediatrics. 2016;**138**:e20160123

[13] American Academy of Pediatrics. Health supervision for children with Down syndrome. American Academy of Pediatrics. 2001;**107**:442-449

[14] Dennis J, Archer N, Ellis J, et al. Recognising heart disease in children with Down syndrome. Archives of Disease in Childhood – Education and Practice. 2010;**95**:98-104

[15] Wren C, Richmond S, Donaldson L, et al. Presentation of congenital heart disease in infancy: Implications for routine examination. Archives of Disease in Childhood. Fetal and Neonatal Edition. 1999;**80**:F49-F53

[16] Craig B. Atrioventricular septal defect: From fetus to adult. Heart. 2006;**92**:1879-1885

[17] Frid C, Drott P, Lundell B, et al. Mortality in Down's syndrome in relation to congenital malformations. Journal of Intellectual Disability Research. 1999;**43**:234-241

[18] Stoll C, Dott B, Alembik Y, et al. Associated congenital anomalies among cases with Down syndrome. European Journal of Medical Genetics. 2015;**58**:674-680

[19] Calkoen EE, Hazekamp MGG, Blom NA, et al. Atrioventricular septal defect: From embryonic development to long term follow up. International Journal of Cardiology. 2016;**202**:784-795

[20] Cohen MS. Common atrioventricular canal defects. In: Lai WW, Mertens LL, Cohen MS, Geva T, editors. Echocardiography in Pediatrics and Congenital Heart Disease: From Fetus to Adult. United Kingdom: Wiley-Blackwell Publishing; 2009

[21] Vergara P, Digilio MC, Zorzi AD, et al. Genetic heterogeneity and phenotypic anomalies in children with atrioventricular canal defect and tetralogy of Fallot. Clinical Dysmorphology. 2006;**15**:65-70

[22] Rizzoli G, Mazzucco A, Maizza F, et al. Does Down syndrome affect prognosis of surgically managed atrioventricular canal defects? The Journal of Thoracic and Cardiovascular Surgery. 1992;**105**:945-953

[23] Masuda M, Kado H, Tanoue Y, et al. Does Down syndrome affect the longterm results of complete atrioventricular septal defect when the defect is repaired during the first year of life? European Journal of Cardio-Thoracic Surgery. 2005;**27**:405-409

[24] NICOR website. Available from: https://nicor4.nicor.org.uk/CHD/an_paeds.nsf/vwContent/home. [Accessed: Aug 27, 2017]

[25] Berger TJ, Blackstone EH, Kirklin JW, et al. Survival and probability of cure with and without operation in complete atrioventricular canal. The Annals of Thoracic Surgery. 1979;**27**:104-111

[26] Najim HK, Coles JG, Endo M et al. Complete atrioventricular septal defects: results of repair, risk factors and freedom from reoperation. Circulation. 1997;**96**:II-311-315

[27] El-Najdawi EK, Driscoll DJ, Puga FJ, et al. Operation for partial atrioventricular septal defect: A forty year review. The Journal of Thoracic and Cardiovascular Surgery. 2000;**199**:880-890

[28] Srivastava S, Parness IA. Tetralogy of Fallot. In: Lai WW, Mertens LL, Cohen MS, Geva T, editors. Echocardiography in Pediatrics and Congenital Heart Disease: From Fetus to Adult. United Kingdom: Wiley-Blackwell Publishing; 2009

[29] Downing TE, Kim YY. Tetralogy of Fallot: General principles of management. Cardiology Clinics. 2015;**33**:531-541

[30] Sullivan RT, Frommelt PC, Hill GD. Earlier pulmonary valve replacement in Down syndrome patients following tetralogy of Fallot repair. Pediatric Cardiology. 2017;**38**: 1251-1256

[31] Forbus GA, Shirali GS. Anomalies of the ventricular septum. In: Lai WW, Mertens LL, Cohen MS, Geva T, editors. Echocardiography in Pediatrics and Congenital Heart Disease: From Fetus to Adult. United Kingdom: Wiley-Blackwell Publishing; 2009

[32] Marino B, Papa M, Guccione P, et al. Ventricular septal defects in Down syndrome. Anatomic types and associated malformations. American Journal of Diseases of Children. 1990;**144**:544-545

[33] D'Alto M, Mahadevan VS. Pulmonary arterial hypertension associated with congenital heart disesase. European Respiratory Review. 2012;**21**:328-337

[34] Cappelli-Bigazzi M, Santoro G, Battaglia C, et al. Endothelial cell function in patients with Down's syndrome. The American Journal of Cardiology. 2004;**94**:392-395

[35] Van de Bruaene A, Delcroix M, Pasuet A, et al. The Belgian Eisenmenger syndrome registry: Implications for treatment strategies? Acta Cardiologica. 2009;**64**:447-453

Chapter 7

Mitochondrial Abnormalities in Down Syndrome: Pathogenesis, Effects and Therapeutic Approaches

Antonella Izzo, Nunzia Mollo, Rita Cicatiello,
Rita Genesio, Simona Paladino, Anna Conti and
Lucio Nitsch

Additional information is available at the end of the chapter

http://dx.doi.org/10.5772/intechopen.71059

Abstract

Down syndrome (DS) consists of a complex phenotype with constant features, such as mental retardation and hypotonia, and variable features, including heart defects and susceptibility to Alzheimer's disease, type 2 diabetes, obesity and immune disorders. Overexpression of genes mapping to chromosome 21 (Hsa21) is directly or indirectly responsible for pathogenesis of DS phenotypic features, as overexpressed Hsa21 genes dysregulate several other genes mapping to different chromosomes. Many of these genes are involved in mitochondrial function. Recent studies highlight a link between mitochondrial dysfunction, consistently observed in DS subjects, and DS phenotype. In this review, we first provide a basic overview of mitochondrial alterations in DS in terms of mitochondrial bioenergetics, biogenesis and morphology. We then discuss how mitochondrial malfunction may contribute to the pathogenesis of clinical manifestations and how specific Hsa21 genes may cause the disruption of mitochondrial phenotype. Finally, we focus on drugs, which affect mitochondrial function and network to propose possible therapeutic approaches aimed at improving and/or preventing various aspects of the DS phenotype. Our working hypothesis is that correcting the mitochondrial defect might improve the neurological phenotype and prevent DS-associated pathologies, thus providing a better quality of life for DS individuals and their families.

Keywords: Down syndrome, trisomy 21, mitochondrial dysfunction, mitochondrial dynamics, Down syndrome/therapy

1. Introduction

Down syndrome (DS) (OMIM 190685), caused by the trisomy of chromosome 21 (TS21), is the most common autosomal aneuploidy compatible with postnatal survival with a prevalence of

1 in 700 newborns. Its phenotype is highly complex showing constant features, such as mental retardation, dysmorphic traits and hypotonia, and variable features, including heart defects, susceptibility to Alzheimer's disease (AD), type 2 diabetes, obesity and immune disorders. DS is also a risk factor for a number of diseases, such as thyroid dysfunction, leukemia and various other congenital malformations. The mechanisms causing the DS phenotype are still largely unknown and little progress has been registered so far in the therapeutic approach to ameliorate the life of DS subjects.

Overexpression of genes mapping to chromosome 21 (Hsa21) is clearly responsible for pathogenesis of DS phenotypic features either in a direct or indirect manner, as overexpressed Hsa21 genes affect the regulation of several other genes mapping to different chromosomes. Many of these genes are involved in oxidative phosphorylation (OXPHOS) and more generally in the mitochondrial function [1].

As fully described in the following paragraphs, the mitochondrial dysfunction together with the disruption of the mitochondrial network might concur to determine DS phenotypic traits. This suggests that correcting the mitochondrial defect might affect the severity of DS phenotype.

This review provides first a basic overview of mitochondrial alterations in terms of mitochondrial bioenergetics, biogenesis and morphology in DS. The latest theories are reported about: (i) how mitochondrial malfunction may contribute to the pathogenesis of clinical manifestations of DS and (ii) how specific Hsa21 genes may be involved in determining the pathogenesis of mitochondrial dysfunction in DS. Finally, we focus on drugs that target genes and/or pathways involved in mitochondrial function and mitochondrial network to examine potential therapeutic approaches.

2. Mitochondrial abnormalities in DS

Increasing evidences, widely documented in scientific literature, highlight that there is a link between mitochondrial damages and the complex DS phenotype. The downregulation of nuclear-encoded mitochondrial genes (NEMGs) is a hallmark of TS21 in human fetal hearts [1] and brains [2]. Transcriptome analysis of fetal heart tissues showed that more than 400 genes located on chromosomes other than 21 were differentially expressed, either upregulated or downregulated, in trisomic versus non-trisomic hearts [1]. Functional class scoring of these genes revealed a global downregulation of NEMGs. Together with the downregulation of genes involved in mitochondrial pathways, we demonstrated, in trisomic fetal fibroblasts of the same subjects, that mitochondria exhibited morphological abnormalities like increased size, irregular shape and evident breaks, mainly of inner membranes. Mitochondria with concentric and longitudinal cristae were significantly more abundant. Stereological analysis demonstrated that mean mitochondrial volume was significantly lower in DS cells [3, 4]. All indices of mitochondrial respiratory functions were decreased and a significant alteration in the redox homeostasis was observed, highlighted by an increased production of reactive oxygen species (ROS) and a higher steady level of intra-mitochondrial Ca^{2+} [3]. DS fibroblasts also showed a deficit of whole energy status as demonstrated by a decrease of basal ATP content and of mitochondrial membrane potential (**Figure 1**) [4].

Representative confocal microscopy live cell imaging of TMRM fluorescence in euploid and trisomic fibroblasts. A significant decrease in fluorescence intensity is observed in trisomic samples when compared with euploid ones.

These results were in agreement with different studies that demonstrated a less efficient mitochondrial energy production apparatus in fibroblasts from DS subjects due to the impairment of mitochondrial respiratory chain complex I, ATP synthase, ADP/ATP translocator and adenylate kinase activities [5, 6].

The protein expression of mitochondrial electron transport enzyme subunits has been found decreased in the brain of people affected by DS [7]. Decreased mitochondrial redox activity and membrane potential have also been observed both in DS astrocytes [8, 9] and in the brain of the Ts1Cje mouse model [10]. In neural progenitor cells (NPCs) isolated from the hippocampus of Ts65Dn mice, another widely used model of DS, a severe impairment of mitochondrial bioenergetics and biogenesis and reduced NPCs proliferation were demonstrated [11]. Furthermore, microarray analysis revealed that numerous pathways were altered in Ts65Dn muscle, including pathways involved in ATP biosynthesis [12].

Together with mitochondrial function alterations, a significant disruption of mitochondrial dynamics has been observed in trisomic cells. An increased fragmentation of the mitochondrial network was demonstrated in primary cultures of TS21 astrocytes and neurons [13] and in trisomic fetal fibroblasts [4] (**Figure 2**). In agreement with the impairment of mitochondrial network towards the fragmentation, the expression of *MFN2* and *OPA1*, two fusion-inducing genes, was decreased in the same cells.

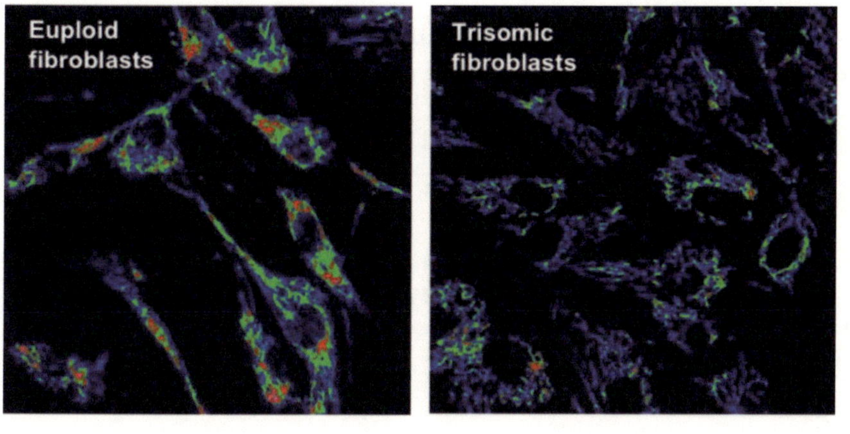

Figure 1. A significant decrease of fluorescence intensity demonstrates that membrane potential is reduced in DS fibroblasts.

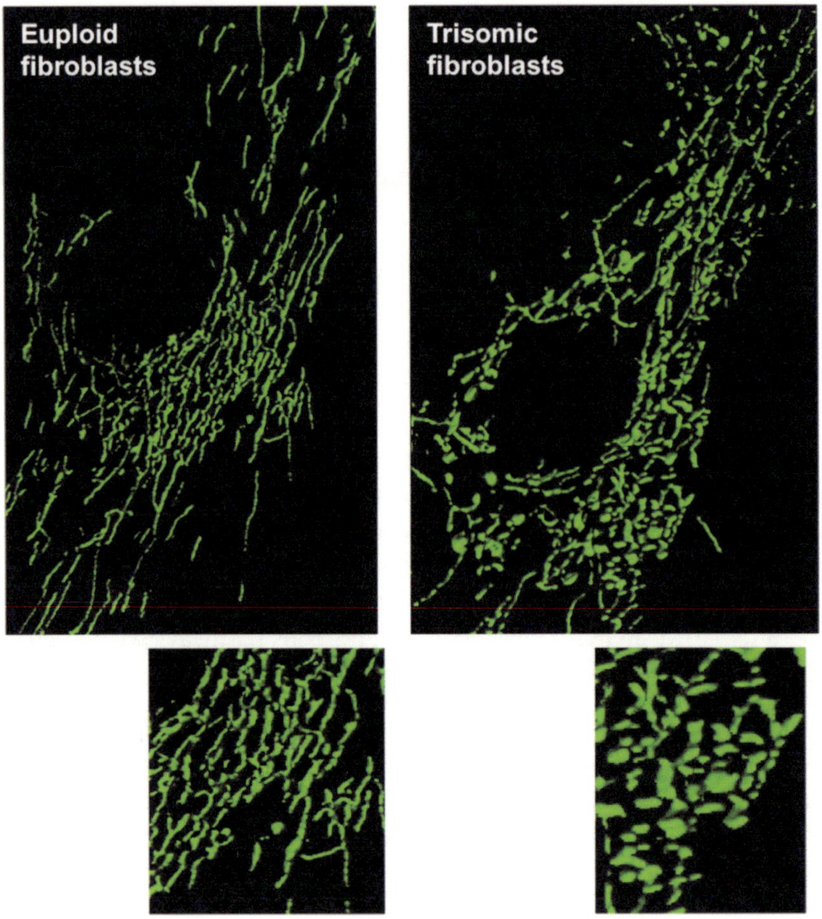

Figure 2. Mitochondrial network is fragmented in DS fibroblasts.

Representative images showing that the mitochondrial network is less fragmented in euploid fibroblasts than in trisomic ones. Magnifications of intracellular selected details show that the number of mitochondria is significantly higher in trisomic cells compared with non-trisomic cells.

A link between mitophagy and mitochondrial dynamics has been recently demonstrated [14, 15], as mitochondrial fusion and fission play a significant role in disease-related processes, such as mitophagy and apoptosis. Dysfunctional and damaged mitochondria are removed from the mitochondrial network via mitophagy processes. The segregation of impaired mitochondria due either to fission or to inhibition of fusion mechanism is hypothesized to be a requirement for this mitophagic degradation [16]. Mitophagy impairments are involved in the development of several neurodegenerative diseases [17].

The knowledge of molecular bases of mitochondrial dysfunction is allowing to set-up most appropriate therapeutic solutions to counteract it, as more fully described in the following paragraphs.

3. Pathogenesis of mitochondrial dysfunction in DS

3.1. *PGC-1α* is a key modulator of mitochondrial biogenesis and respiratory function

A common denominator of most of the events that affect mitochondrial function is the transcriptional coactivator *PGC-1α/PPARGC-1α* (peroxisome proliferator-activated receptor gamma coactivator 1alpha), a master regulator of mitochondrial activity [4–6]. *PGC-1α*, through the interaction with transcriptional partners, such as *NRF1*, *ERRa*, *PPARs* and *YY1*, promotes mitochondrial biogenesis and regulates mitochondrial respiratory capacity [18, 19]. Also these *PGC-1α* transcriptional partners, as well as many NEMGs, have been found downregulated in DS fetal heart tissue [1] and fibroblasts [3]. *PGC-1α* knockout mice manifest a reduction of mitochondrial number and of respiratory capacity in skeletal muscle [18].

PGC-1α transcription and activity are positively regulated by Ca^{2+} signaling and negatively regulated by the Hsa21-coded corepressor *NRIP1* (nuclear receptor interacting protein 1) [19]. Indeed, *PGC-1α* has been found hypoexpressed at the transcriptional and protein levels in TS21 fetal fibroblasts, directly correlated with the amount of mtDNA, while *NRIP1* was upregulated [3]. PGC-1α activity was also found decreased in the hippocampus of DS patients, as well as in Alzheimer's, Huntington's (HD) and Parkinson's (PD) disease patients [20].

3.2. Role of Hsa21 genes in mitochondrial dysfunction

Little is known about the mechanisms by which trisomy 21 causes the abnormal features typical of the DS phenotype, apart the knowledge that the dosage imbalance of genes on Hsa21 and the resulting dysregulation of genes mapping to different chromosomes share the responsibility for molecular dysfunctions in DS.

Hsa21 gene expression was found globally upregulated 1.5-fold in trisomic samples [1, 2], in full agreement with a gene-dosage effect. A comprehensive meta-analysis from 45 DS gene expression studies [21] identified 77 Hsa21 genes mostly upregulated across all the studies, which are likely involved in the DS phenotype. Six of the genes included in this list, namely *NRIP1*, *SUMO3*, *DYRK1A*, *DSCR1/RCAN1*, *SOD1* and *APP*, are directly or indirectly involved in mitochondrial function. Other Hsa21 genes not included in the Vilardell's list, such as *ETS-2*, *ITSN1*, *PKNOX1/PREP1*, *BACH1* and S100B, were found to be involved in apoptotic events and/or to contribute to the regulation of oxidative stress when overexpressed [22]. The dysregulation of one or more of these genes, listed in **Table 1**, might account for mitochondrial alterations observed in DS, as discussed below.

3.2.1. NRIP1

We recently demonstrated that *NRIP1* overexpression is responsible for decreased respiratory efficiency and altered morphology of mitochondria in DS [23]. *NRIP1* is a corepressor that interacts with nuclear receptors and regulates the expression of genes that control metabolic processes such as energy homeostasis [24–27]. Its activity on mitochondrial pathways is

Genes and transcripts	Effects on mitochondrial phenotype
NRIP1/RIP140—nuclear receptor interacting protein 1	Decreases respiratory efficiency and alters morphology of mitochondria
APP—amyloid beta precursor protein	Induces mitochondrial oxidative stress and mitochondrial dysfunction
SUMO3—small ubiquitin-like modifier 3	Modulates *NRIP1* repressive activity and attenuates the transcriptional activity of *PGC-1α*
DYRK1A—dual-specificity tyrosine phosphorylation-regulated kinase 1A	Controls *PGC-1α* via the *calcineurin/NFAT* pathway
DSCR1/RCAN1—Down Syndrome critical region gene 1	Controls *PGC-1α* via the *calcineurin/NFAT* pathway and is associated with calcium overloading
SOD1—superoxide dismutase 1	Is associated with oxidative stress
ETS-2—V-ETS avian erythroblastosis virus E26 oncogene homolog 2	Promotes the activation of a mitochondrial death pathway
ITSN1—Intersectin 1	Regulates the mitochondrial apoptotic pathway
PREP1—PBX-regualting protein 1	Inhibits the OXPHOS negatively regulating *PGC-1α* and mitochondrial fusion genes *OPA1* and *MFN2*
BACH1—BTB domain and CNC homolog 1	Contributes to the early increase of oxidative stress in DS through the inhibition of the *HO-1/BVR-A* axis
S100B—S100 calcium-binding protein, beta	Overexpression induces ROS formation, activation of stress response kinases and increased programmed cell death
hsa-mir-155	Affects mitochondrial biogenesis by targeting *TFAM*
hsa-let-7c	May affect mitochondrial function by targeting *ANT1*

Table 1. Hsa21 genes and transcripts involved in mitochondrial function.

mainly exerted through the repressive control of *PGC-1α* [19]; the two proteins have mutually antagonizing roles in NEMG regulation. In neonatal rat cardiomyocytes, it was demonstrated that overexpressed *NRIP1* abrogates *PGC-1α*-mediated induction of mitochondrial membrane potential and mitochondrial biogenesis [25]. Furthermore, at least 1/3 of NEMGs upregulated after *PGC-1α* induction in human osteoblast-like cells [28] were found to be *NRIP1* targets [23].

To assess that, among the Hsa21 transcription regulators, *NRIP1* was indeed the main dysregulator of mitochondrial gene expression, the Gene Expression Omnibus (GEO) repository (http://www.ncbi.nlm.nih.gov/geo) was screened for gene expression data related to the modulation of Hsa21 genes. The functional class scoring of the lists of genes dysregulated, when Hsa21 genes were individually overexpressed (GSE19836 experiment [29]), demonstrated that, among the Hsa21 transcription factors or regulators, only *NRIP1* was able to affect NEMG regulation with a cluster of 37 NEMGs downregulated after *NRIP1* overexpression [23].

We then demonstrated that *NRIP1* attenuation by siRNA in DS fibroblasts affected NEMG expression, increased *PGC-1α* expression and counteracted mitochondrial dysfunction in terms of ROS production, mitochondrial activity, mitochondrial calcium and ATP content [23].

These findings indicate that the Hsa21 gene *NRIP1* strongly contributes to the mitochondrial dysfunction observed in DS and suggest that the *NRIP1-PGC-1α* axis might represent a potential therapeutic target for restoring altered mitochondrial function in DS.

3.2.2. APP

Mitochondrial abnormalities and a decreased COX activity might also be induced by overproduction of beta-*APP* [30], although the TS1Cje mouse model, in which *APP* is not triplicated, also shows decreased mitochondrial function and ATP production [10]. Overexpression of APP induces mitochondrial oxidative stress and activates the intrinsic apoptotic cascade [31]. In addition, amyloid-β fragments, particularly Aβ42, exert direct toxic effects on cells, including Ca^{2+} dysregulation, mitochondrial dysfunction and induction of oxidative stress [32, 33]. APP protein has been demonstrated to progressively accumulate within mitochondrial matrix leading to increased free radicals and impaired mitochondrial metabolism [34]. In addition, APP have been shown to translocate into mitochondria when overexpressed in a human cortical neuronal cell line [35]. *APP* exerts synergistic effects with other Hsa21 genes [36].

3.2.3. SUMO3

It may affect mitochondrial function by modulating the *NRIP1* repressive activity [37]. SUMOylation also attenuates the transcriptional activity of *PGC-1α*, possibly by enhancing the interaction between *PGC-1α* and the corepressor *NRIP1* that alters its nuclear distribution [38]. *SUMO3* overexpression in DS could therefore be responsible for a concurrent improvement of *NRIP1* function and decrease of *PGC-1α* activity.

3.2.4. DYRK1A and DSCR1/RCAN1

The protein products of these genes interact functionally. Their increased dosage cooperatively leads to dysregulation of the signaling pathways that are controlled by *NFAT* family of transcription factors, with potential consequences for several organs and systems that are affected in DS individuals [39]. The two genes control *PGC-1α* activity via the calcineurin/NFAT pathway [40], namely through the binding of *NFATc* genes to the *PGC-1α* promoter [41]. Calcineurin is involved in the regulation of many cellular processes, including cardiac hypertrophy, skeletal-muscle development, synaptic plasticity and T-cell activation [39].

RCAN1, also known as calcipressin, has been found chronically overexpressed in the brain of both DS patients and sporadic AD patients [42]. *RCAN1* overexpression has been linked to oxidative stress and mitochondrial dysfunction [42–45] and is strictly related to calcium overloading [46], as it affects mitochondrial permeability transition pore (mPTP) function. *RCAN1*-induced mPTP opening leads to a series of consequences, including Ca^{2+} retention incapability, massive swelling of mitochondria and rupture of the outer membrane [46]. In agreement with these data, deregulation of Ca^{2+} homeostasis and Ca^{2+}-mediated signaling has been described in cells derived from trisomic patients or in murine models of DS [47]. Mitochondrial Ca^{2+} concentration was found significantly higher in fibroblasts from DS feti [3], which also show swelled mitochondria with damaged membranes [4].

The overexpression of the brain-specific *RCAN1.1S* isoform in mice promotes dysregulation of dynamin-related protein 1 (*DRP1*), a protein that promotes mitochondrial fission [48]. Accordingly, *RCAN1* was found to induce mitochondrial autophagy in cardiomyocytes [49].

3.2.5. *SOD1*

The redox imbalance in DS has been long attributed to overexpression of Cu/Zn superoxide dismutase *SOD1*, whose levels are approximately 50% greater in cells from DS patients than in normal ones [50]. *SOD1*, the major *SOD* in mammalian cells, catalyzes the dismutation of superoxide radicals to H_2O_2 and O_2 and is an important antioxidant defense system [51].

3.2.6. *ETS-2*

Studies in transgenic mice showed that *ETS-2* overexpression induces apoptosis of thymus, spleen and brain cells [52]. Furthermore, ETS-2 promotes the activation of a mitochondrial death pathway in DS neurons. Overexpression of *ETS-2* induces cytochrome c translocation to the cytoplasm and apoptotic features in normal human cortical neurons [53].

3.2.7. *ITSN1*

This gene regulates the mitochondrial apoptotic pathway in endothelial cells [54].

3.2.8. *PKNOX1/PREP1*

This gene, which encodes for a homeodomain transcription factor, is involved in embryonic development regulating the homeobox protein Pbx activity [55]. DS human fibroblasts that express higher levels of *PREP1* are more sensitive to genotoxic stress. *PREP1* demonstrated to regulate mitochondrial oxidative phosphorylation components. It directly binds to the promoter region of genes encoding mitochondrial components [56] and indirectly controls the stability of p160 Myb-binding protein, a powerful negative regulator of *PGC-1α* activity [57]. In the muscle of *Prep1* ablated mice, *Pgc-1α* expression was increased with consequent increasing in abundance of mitochondrial OXPHOS proteins and in citrate synthase activity together with an improved maximal oxidative capacity. Most important, Prep1 ablation significantly increased the abundance of *Opa1* and *Mfn2*, two genes inducing mitochondrial fusion [56]. These results suggest that *PREP1* negatively regulates OXPHOS and mitochondrial network.

3.2.9. *BACH1*

This gene is a transcriptional regulator, which acts as hypoxia regulator by binding to antioxidant response elements of DNA thus inhibiting the transcription of specific genes involved in cell stress response, including heme oxygenase-1 (HO-1). HO-1 and its partner, biliverdin reductase-A (BVR-A), are upregulated in response to oxidative stress. BACH1 protein was found decreased in DS brains, coupled with reduced induction of brain HO-1. This supports the hypothesis that the dysregulation of HO-1/BVR-A system contributes to the early increase of oxidative stress in DS and provides potential mechanistic pathways involved in the neurodegenerative process and AD development [58].

3.2.10. S100B

This gene codes for the b subunit of S100 proteins, a large family of calcium-binding proteins. The S100B homodimer is the major form in the mammalian brain. It can stimulate neurite extension [59] and plays a role in synaptogenesis [60], dendritic branching [61] and apoptosis [62]. S100B protein has long been suggested to be involved in glial cell activation and neuroinflammation [63]. Elevated brain *S100B* expression occurs in various disease states, including AD and DS. *S100B* plays an important role in neuroinflammation and in the regulation and maintenance of the serotonergic nervous system, with a particular focus on the hippocampus [64].

In vitro studies of DS fetal human neural precursors (HNP) demonstrated that *S100B* is constitutively overexpressed in these cells and that overexpression leads to increased ROS formation, activation of stress response kinases and increased programmed cell death. Further studies demonstrated that DS HNPs adopt more gliocentric progenitor phenotypes, if compared with euploid controls, with a consequent reduction in neuronogenesis [65].

3.3. Hsa21 miRNAs involved in mitochondrial phenotype

Hsa21 encodes several classes of non-coding RNAs, the most enriched being long non-coding RNAs, while miRNAs are the less represented [66]. The most recent annotation of miRNA database (miRBase, release 21) reports 29 miRNAs mapping to Hsa21. At least two of them, miR-155-5p and let-7c-5p, are possibly involved in mitochondrial function.

It was recently reported that the Hsa21 miR-155-5p affects mitochondrial biogenesis by targeting the mitochondrial transcription factor A (*TFAM*) [67], a gene that was found downregulated in trisomic hearts [1]. TFAM is a nuclear-encoded protein that controls the transcription and maintenance of mtDNA and therefore mitochondrial biogenesis.

Another Hsa21 miRNA potential candidate for mitochondrial anomalies is let-7c. By bioinformatics analysis, it appears to have several targets among genes that were found downregulated in trisomic fetal hearts and involved in mitochondrial function. Among these targets, *SLC25A4/ANT1* [68] appeared as a potential candidate for both mitochondrial dysfunction and congenital heart defects in DS. This gene functions as a gated pore that translocates ADP and ATP between cytoplasm and mitochondria, regulating the intracellular energetic balance. Furthermore, its dysregulation has been associated to mitochondrial cardiomyopathies [69] and its genetic inactivation results in mtDNA damage and ROS increase [8].

4. How mitochondrial dysfunction might affect DS clinical phenotype?

4.1. Muscle hypotonia

DS patients suffer from muscle hypotonia and altered motor coordination. In theTs65Dn mice, the ultrastructural analysis of myofibrils showed mitochondrial structural changes [12, 70], whereas microarray analysis revealed that pathways involved in ATP biosynthesis, proteolysis, glucose and fat metabolism and neuromuscular transmission were dysregulated [12].

Skeletal muscle is particularly vulnerable to oxidative stress. The disruption of mitochondrial network towards fragmentation, together with mitochondrial dysfunction, is an essential step of the muscular atrophy programme in adult animals [71]. Conversely, inhibition of the mitochondrial fission inhibits muscle loss [72]. Furthermore, changes in mitochondrial morphology have been implicated in apoptosis as well as in the regulation of muscle metabolism [73].

It is worth noting that patients with DS have features of premature aging [74, 75] and exhibit a decrement in muscle strength if compared with euploid subjects, similar to what occurs in aged versus young persons [76]. It is, therefore, possible that muscle hypotonia and motor dysfunction in DS share some basic mechanisms with the progressive age-related decrease in skeletal muscle mass, strength and quality known as sarcopenia [77].

4.2. Intellectual disability and neurodegeneration

Increasing evidences are demonstrating that mitochondrial function is a key actor in the events that lead to intellectual disability and neurodegeneration in DS. Development of the DS brain is associated with decreased neuronal number and abnormal neuronal differentiation [78]. Patients with DS show higher levels of oxidative stress at all ages and apoptosis and generation of ROS are increased in human fetal DS neurons if compared with the general population [78, 79]. DS astrocytes and neuronal cultures [8, 9] as well as the brain of the Ts1Cje mouse model [10] show a decrease of mitochondrial membrane potential, ATP production and an increase of reactive oxygen species [10]. Mitochondrial bioenergetics and biogenesis are impaired during neural progenitor cell (NPC) proliferation in Ts65Dn cells [11]. Mitochondrial morphology was found consistently altered in TS21 astrocytes and neurons, which exhibit increased fragmentation of the mitochondrial network [13]. Mitochondrial function, fission-fusion mechanisms, biogenesis and degradation are critical for synaptogenesis, Ca^{2+} buffering, axonal transport and bioenergetics [80]. Functionally and structurally damaged mitochondria do not produce sufficient ATP and are more prone in producing pro-apoptotic factors and ROS [81], which also represent an early stage in neurodegenerative process [82]. An increased risk for AD manifests in most of DS individuals starting from 40 years of age [83, 84]. The similarity of neurodegenerative processes between DS and Alzheimer disease (AD) and the high prevalence of AD in DS patients suggest that AD and DS share common brain alterations possibly due to similar molecular pathways involved in the pathogenesis, such as mitochondrial dysfunction and oxidative stress [85]. Energy depletion and

http://dx.doi.org/10.5772/intechopen.71059

oxidative stress can also induce amyloidogenic changes in AβPP processing [86]. Busciglio et al. [9] demonstrated that there is a marked alteration in AβPP processing and Aβ trafficking in cortical DS astrocytes and neurons, similar to those induced in normal human astrocytes by inhibition of mitochondrial energy metabolism.

It is important to note that neurodegenerative diseases, such as AD, PD and HD, show alterations of mitochondrial function and fusion and/or fission processes very similar to those observed in DS [82, 87] as well as a similar dysregulation of mitochondria-related genes most of which are target of the *NRIP1/PGC-1α* axis [23].

4.3. Heart defects

DS is a major cause of congenital heart defects (CHD), mostly derived from endocardial cushion anomalies, such as atrioventricular septal defects, ventricular septal defects and tetralogy of Fallot [88, 89].

Transcriptome analysis of human fetal heart tissues from DS subjects has shown a global significant downregulation of NEMGs. Genes from all five complexes were downregulated, suggesting that the corresponding proteins and enzymatic activities might be reduced and that the mitochondrial function could be consequently impaired [1]. When mitochondrial phenotype was analyzed in fibroblasts from the same subjects, a more pronounced chronic pro-oxidative state was demonstrated in DS fetuses with congenital heart defects if compared with feti without cardiopathy [3]. Significant differences in mitochondrial respiration, complex I activity and ROS production were observed, suggesting a relationship between mitochondrial function and cardiac phenotype [3]. These alterations might be harbingers of the heart defects associated with Hsa21 trisomy, which could be based on elusive mechanisms involving genetic variability, environmental factors and/or stochastic events [1].

Searching for a link between heart development and mitochondria, the focus falls on the Hsa21 genes *DYRK1A* and *RCAN1*, which play a role in the calcineurin/NFAT pathway [40] and are believed to affect both mitochondrial activity and morphology during heart development [90, 91]. *DYRK1A* and *RCAN1* are involved in regulating the levels of NFATc phosphorylation. The calcineurin/NFAT signaling pathway is known to be a critical regulator of organogenesis [92] and the NFATc transcription factors are transiently expressed in the endocardial cushions during heart septation [91]. The *DSCR1* and *DYRK1A* genes, both mapping on Hsa21 within the critical region for DS, act synergistically to prevent nuclear translocation of *NFATc* transcription factors and may cause their downregulation [40]. Even modest overexpression of *DYRK1A* decreases NFATc protein activity and levels and may induce vascular and cardiac defects [40]. The inhibition of the mitochondrial activity in Nfatc3$^{-/-}$Nfatc4$^{-/-}$ cardiomyocytes [90] suggests that the calcineurin/NFAT pathway affects mitochondrial activity during heart development. *Nfatc*-null mice show phenotypic anomalies that resemble those observed in human DS and 65% of *Nfat*c1–4-null mice have endocardial cushion defects [40]. In human DS fetal fibroblasts and hearts, *NFAT*c3 and *NFAT*c4 were found significantly downregulated, whereas *DYRK1A* and *RCAN1* were overexpressed possibly due to dosage effect [1, 3].

In addition to congenital heart defects, DS subject may develop ventricular hypertrophy during the post-natal life possibly as a result of reduced mitochondrial electron-transport chain activity and oxygen consumption. Alterations in mitochondrial function observed in right ventricular cardiac hypertrophy are mainly attributed to complex I dysfunction [93]. *NRIP1*-dependent repression of mitochondria related genes may be involved in the pathogenesis of this defect. The overexpression of this gene in a transgenic mouse demonstrated to cause cardiac hypertrophy [94].

Also the Hsa21 miR-155, a known repressor of *TFAM* gene [67], was uncovered as an inducer of pathological cardiomyocyte hypertrophy, suggesting that inhibition of endogenous miR-155 might have clinical potential to suppress cardiac hypertrophy and heart failure [95]. MiR-155 is overexpressed in fetal heart tissue possibly due to dosage effect [68].

4.4. Type 2 diabetes and obesity

Children with DS have an increased risk of developing endocrine disorders such as type 2 diabetes and obesity [96]. The hypothesis that prominent features of type 2 diabetes and the condition of obesity are caused by mitochondrial dysfunction and by an impaired bioenergetics capacity is definitively emerging [97]. Given the important role that mitochondria play for bioenergetics support of signal transduction, fat oxidation and substrate transport, an impairment of electron transport chain activity may have particular relevance to the pathogenesis of insulin resistance in type 2 diabetes [98]. This hypothesis is substantiated by two evidences: (i) a disproportionately large reduction of electron transport chain activity has been observed in the subsarcolemmal mitochondrial fraction in type 2 diabetic and obese subjects if compared with unaffected volunteers and (ii) mitochondria from human skeletal muscle were found to be smaller and to have reduced activity of complex I in both type 2 diabetes and obesity [99].

Interestingly, the Hsa21 corepressor gene *NRIP1* and its target *PGC-1α* play key roles in the transcriptional regulation of genes involved in energy homeostasis. The expression and promoter activity of CIDEA, an important regulatory factor in adipose cell function and obesity, is repressed by *NRIP1* and induced by *PGC-1α* [100]. These genes are also involved in glucose uptake by affecting the regulation of both transcription and subcellular localization of the insulin-sensitive glucose transporter *GLUT4* [101]. This evidence suggested that *NRIP1* might be a potential therapeutic target in the treatment of insulin resistance in obese and type 2 diabetic patients [101]. Accordingly, mice lacking *Nrip1* are lean, show resistance to high-fat diet-induced obesity and have increased oxygen consumption [102].

Some evidences support the role of an altered mitochondrial dynamics in obesity. It is known that obesity in both humans and mice is associated with reduced *Mfn2* expression and therefore with a defective mitochondrial fusion machinery [103]. Furthermore, an altered proteolytic processing of the GTPase *OPA1* in humans is associated with insulin resistance [104].

4.5. Immune disorders

Children with DS demonstrate an increased susceptibility to infections, usually of the upper respiratory tract [105–107], and autoimmune disorders, including hypothyroidism [108] and celiac disease [109, 110]. The abnormalities of the immune system associated with DS include alteration of B and T-cell number, with marked decrease of naive lymphocytes; abnormal thymus functions and development; impaired mitogen-induced T cell proliferation; reduced specific antibody responses to immunizations and defects of neutrophil chemotaxis [111, 112]. The rates of lymphocyte respiration in the children with DS were found slower than in the control group [113].

Important roles of mitochondrial dynamics in the immune system physiopathology have been recently demonstrated. The first evidence is that mitochondria transportation during lymphocyte migration requires mitochondrial fission [114]. The second is that mitochondrial remodeling works as a signaling mechanism that instructs T cell metabolic programming [115]. This theory arises from the demonstration that T effector (TE) cells show a fragmented network with punctuate mitochondria, whereas T memory (TM) cells show fused networks. Accordingly, in transgenic Opa1$^{-/-}$ mice, TM lymphocytes show a decreased survival associated with altered cristae structure and decreased spare respiratory capacity. In addition, TE cells could be shifted to a TM fate depending upon changes of mitochondrial dynamics. These data suggest that, by altering cristae morphology, fusion in TM cells configures electron transport chain (ETC) complex associations favoring OXPHOS and fatty acid oxidation, whereas fission in TE cells leads to cristae expansion, reducing ETC efficiency and promoting aerobic glycolysis [115].

5. Therapeutic approaches to improve mitochondrial function in DS

5.1. Possible therapeutic targets

As mitochondrial dysfunction might concur to determine DS mental retardation and other health problems, we might expect that counteracting the mitochondrial defects will improve and/or prevent some aspects of the DS phenotype.

The few clinical trials so far undertaken to restore mitochondrial function in DS subjects using antioxidants and nutraceutics have yielded either poor or discordant outcomes [116, 117]. Better results were obtained on learning and memory in the mouse model Ts65Dn using pentylenetetrazole, memantine, fluoxetine, lithium, epigallocatechin-3-gallate (EGCG) and antioxidants such as vitamin E [118]. Also in this case, the clinical trials have not yielded the expected results.

The key role of *PGC-1α* as a modulator of mitochondrial biogenesis and respiratory function suggests that therapeutic approach on mitochondrial dysfunction in DS could be based either on *PGC-1α* activators, which have been tested in mouse models for other disease [119–122], or on PPARg agonists, which demonstrated to attenuate mitochondrial dysfunction in AD mouse models [123–126].

It is known that *PGC-1α* activity is mainly controlled by *PPARs*, AMP-activated kinases (*AMPKs*) and the NAD-dependent deacetylase SIRT1 [127]. Direct phosphorylation by AMPK promotes *PGC-1α*-dependent induction at the *PGC-1α* promoter level [122], whereas *SIRT1* stimulates *PGC-1α* activity through deacetylation, thereby inducing mitochondrial biogenesis [119]. Pharmacological activators for these proteins, such as metformin, via *AMPK* induction, and resveratrol, via *SIRT1* induction, have been tested in mouse models for neurodegenerative diseases in which mitochondrial alterations play a central role such as AD, Parkinson's disease and Huntington's disease [120–122].

A comprehensive analysis was performed to evaluate in vitro the effects of potential *PGC-1α* activating drugs [128]. The authors pharmaceutically targeted the PPARs (bezafibrate, rosiglitazone), AMPK (AICAR, metformin) and SIRT1 (resveratrol) pathways in HeLa cells, neuronal cells and *PGC-1α*-deficient MEFs demonstrating tissue-specific effects of these drugs in modulating mitochondrial processes and cellular stress programs. All the observed effects were clearly dependent on *PGC-1α* modulation.

5.2. Advances in preclinical and clinical therapeutic approaches

5.2.1. Antioxidants

Most of the clinical trials so far undertaken in DS patients are based on antioxidant nutrients or vitamin administration to scavenge oxygen-derived free radicals [129, 130].

A study in which a mixture of antioxidants (selenium, zinc, vitamin A, vitamin E and vitamin C) and/or folinic acid was administered as supplementation to children with DS aged under 7 months for about 18 months provided no evidence to support the use of these supplements as this supplementation did not affect oxidative stress [131]. An interesting comment to this study was "This is perhaps not surprising because differences between foetuses with Down's syndrome and unaffected foetuses can be identified after only 11 weeks gestation, implying that by 7 months of age, any damage may already have been done" [132]. Vitamin E administration in a recent study did not demonstrate to slow the progression of cognitive deterioration in older individuals with DS [133].

Coenzyme Q_{10} (CoQ_{10}) is a bioactive quinone ubiquitous in the organism, involved in mitochondrial bioenergetics, with a known role as a lipophilic antioxidant [134]. CoQ_{10} supplementation to 10 patients with TS21 for 3 months demonstrated that the pro-oxidant state in plasma of children with trisomy 21, as assessed by ubiquinol-10:total CoQ_{10} ratio, may be normalized with ubiquinol-10 supplementation [130]. The authors concluded that further studies would be needed to determine whether correction of this oxidant imbalance improves clinical outcomes of children with trisomy 21 but no results in this direction have yet been communicated.

Overall, these results show that antioxidant supplementation is safe but it does neither improve the cognitive performance nor dementia in DS patients.

5.2.2. Melatonin

The antioxidant properties of melatonin induced to study plasma melatonin concentrations in a small group of children with DS [135]. Plasma melatonin concentrations were lower in DS subjects than in age-matched controls. The authors concluded that this constituted an added oxidative risk to children with DS. Melatonin treatment has demonstrated to induce antioxidant and antiaging effects in the hippocampus of adult Ts65Dn mice [136]. Unfortunately, even though this treatment attenuated the oxidative damage and cellular senescence in the brain [136], pre-and post-natal melatonin administration in an additional study partially regulated brain oxidative stress but did not demonstrated to improve cognitive or histological alterations in the same DS mouse model [137].

5.2.3. *Epigallocatechin-3-gallate (EGCG)*

EGCG—a member of a natural polyphenol family—is a mitochondrial-targeted molecule displaying a selective antiapoptotic effect against inducers of mitochondrial oxidative stress in a variety of neuronal cell types [138]. EGCG has been found to prevent mitochondrial deterioration in aged rat brain [139], reduce cerebral amyloidosis [140] and correct amyloid-induced mitochondrial dysfunction in a transgenic mice model of Alzheimer disease [141].

EGCG modulates key regulators of mitochondrial metabolism such as Sirt1 activity [142] and cAMP levels [143, 144] in addition to being a specific and safe inhibitor of the Hsa21 gene *DYRK1A*, a kinase protein involved in brain development and in the control of synaptic plasticity [145]. This makes EGCG an interesting candidate drug for the treatment of DS phenotype.

A therapeutic benefit on mitochondrial activity by EGCG has been demonstrated in cellular and murine model of DS. Indeed EGCG treatment renews the capacity of DS cells to produce energy by mitochondrial OXPHOS and to prevent mitochondrial ROS overproduction [146]. The treatment of neural progenitor cells, isolated from the hippocampus of Ts65Dn, by EGCG reactivates mitochondria bioenergetics and biogenesis and promotes neural progenitor cell proliferation [11]. On the other hand, in vivo studies demonstrated that young adults with DS treated with EGCG exhibit some cognitive benefits, although these effects disappear with time [147]. Furthermore, the treatment carried out in the mouse model Ts65dn in the neonatal period rescues numerous trisomy-linked brain alterations. However, even during this critical time window for hippocampal development, EGCG does not elicit enduring effects on the hippocampal physiology [148].

A further study showed that a temporally specific prenatal EGCG treatment improved some craniofacial dysmorphology associated with DS in Ts65Dn embryos and mice. EGCG in particular improved neural crest cells (NCC)-related deficits in proliferation and migration in vitro in mandibular precursor cells from Ts65Dn E9.5 embryos. In vivo treatment with EGCG at E7 and E8, around the time of the developing NCC deficit, appeared to improve some of the NCC embryonic dysmorphology in Ts65Dn E9.5 embryos [149]. However, a long-lasting EGCG treatment at a lower dose (E0–E9) did not have the same corrective effects.

More recently, the same authors demonstrated that a higher dose of EGCG inTs65Dn mice and euploid littermates failed to improve cognitive deficits; EGCG also produced several detrimental effects on skeleton in both genotypes [150].

In conclusion, EGCG stimulates mitochondrial biogenesis and promotes oxidative phosphorylation through cAMP/PKA- and sirtuin-dependent mechanism [146], and also, at higher concentrations, it promotes apoptosis through mitochondrial damage, membrane depolarization and cytochrome c release [151, 152]. All these results suggest that timing and dosage of EGCG treatment are important and have to be optimized in treating DS-related phenotypes.

5.2.4. Resveratrol

Resveratrol (RSV), a natural polyphenolic compound found in a wide variety of plant species, induces expression of genes involved in mitochondrial biogenesis, oxidative phosphorylation and endogenous antioxidant defense by modulation of cell signaling pathways that control cell homeostasis. RSV treatment protected mice against diet-induced obesity and insulin resistance. This effect was largely explained by an RSV-mediated decrease in *PGC-1α* acetylation and an increase in *PGC-1α* activity [153]. RSV increased the mean life expectancy and maximal lifespan in a mouse model of sporadic and age-related AD. RSV-supplemented animals showed increased Sirt1 expression and consequent downregulation of apoptotic protein p53 in the cortex and hippocampus. Also, p-AMPK in the cortex and total AMPK in the hippocampus were increased [153]. Although thousands of research papers have been published related to RSV pharmacological activities in many diseases, only one study has been performed on the effect of this polyphenol in DS [11]. The authors of the study conclude that RSV can sustain and enhance mitochondrial functions by upregulating *PGC1α*/Sirt1/AMPK axis and promote neural precursor proliferation from Ts65Dn. They suggest resveratrol as a new drug to be tested in vivo as potential therapeutic tool to promote mitochondrial functions, accelerate neurogenesis and ultimately counteract some of the DS clinical features [11].

5.2.5. Metformin

The effects of the biguanide metformin on mitochondrial function have been investigated in human trisomic fibroblasts [4]. Metformin demonstrated to induce both the expression and the activity of *PGC-1α* and to upregulate its target genes *NRF-1* and *TFAM*, thus promoting mitochondrial biogenesis. The drug enhanced ATP production in treated cells and improved overall mitochondrial activity. Most interestingly, metformin treatment counteracted mitochondrial fission observed in trisomic fibroblasts, inducing the formation of a mitochondrial network with a branched and elongated tubular morphology (**Figure 2**) and regulating the expression of genes involved in the fission/fusion machinery, namely *OPA1* and *MFN2* [4].

Metformin has shown to improve cognition in patients with mild cognitive impairment and AD [154]. There were no serious adverse events related to its administration.

Metformin is a drug commonly used as a hypoglycemic agent in type 2 diabetes because it inactivates gluconeogenesis [155]. Metformin activates AMPK in the liver and muscles, causing the phosphorylation and the consequent activation of PGC-1α, and upregulates SIRT1 that in turn activates PGC-1α by deacetylation [155].

Moreover, it has been found that metformin promotes neurogenesis in rodent and human neural precursors and enhances spatial memory formation in normal adult mouse [156].

Metformin is an already registered drug with limited side effects that can be safely administered during pregnancy and crosses both the placental and blood-brain barrier [157, 158]. For these characteristics, it could be immediately introduced in human therapeutic protocols.

6. Conclusions

The study of candidate pathogenic mechanisms in DS is helping scientists to develop more appropriate therapeutic solutions for the treatment of this still untreatable genetic disorder.

A long way has been paved in this direction as we have already gained important knowledge about the importance of bioenergetics mechanisms in determining the DS phenotype and the roles played by Hsa21 genes in this scenario.

The working hypothesis is that counteracting the mitochondrial defect in DS may improve the neurological phenotype and prevent DS-associated pathologies, such as Alzheimer's disease, type 2 diabetes, obesity and hypertrophic cardiopathy, thus providing a better quality of life for DS individuals and their families.

Impaired energy metabolism, defect of mitochondrial enzyme activities and abnormalities of mitochondrial respiration are common characteristics of neurodegenerative conditions [20]. On these premises, restoring the mitochondrial function could represent also a promising strategy to limit the progression of neurodegenerative diseases and even to delay some common aging processes.

Should any of these drugs, already registered for different purposes, demonstrate to be effective, they could be immediately introduced in human therapeutic protocols possibly along with specific therapies aimed at restoring cognitive functions.

Author details

Antonella Izzo, Nunzia Mollo, Rita Cicatiello, Rita Genesio, Simona Paladino, Anna Conti* and Lucio Nitsch

*Address all correspondence to: anconti@unina.it

Department of Molecular Medicine and Medical Biotechnology, University Federico II, Naples, Italy

References

[1] Conti A, Fabbrini F, D'Agostino P, Negri R, Greco D, Genesio R, et al. Altered expression of mitochondrial and extracellular matrix genes in the heart of human fetuses with chromosome 21 trisomy. BMC Genomics. 2007;**8**:268

[2] Mao R, Wang X, Spitznagel EL Jr, Frelin LP, Ting JC, Ding H, et al. Primary and secondary transcriptional effects in the developing human Down syndrome brain and heart. Genome Biology. 2005;**6**(13):R107

[3] Piccoli C, Izzo A, Scrima R, Bonfiglio F, Manco R, Negri R, et al. Chronic pro-oxidative state and mitochondrial dysfunctions are more pronounced in fibroblasts from Down syndrome foeti with congenital heart defects. Human Molecular Genetics. 2013;**22**(6): 1218-1232

[4] Izzo A, Nitti M, Mollo N, Paladino S, Procaccini C, Faicchia D, et al. Metformin restores the mitochondrial network and reverses mitochondrial dysfunction in Down syndrome cells. Human Molecular Genetics. 2017

[5] Valenti D, Tullo A, Caratozzolo MF, Merafina RS, Scartezzini P, Marra E, et al. Impairment of F1F0-ATPase, adenine nucleotide translocator and adenylate kinase causes mitochondrial energy deficit in human skin fibroblasts with chromosome 21 trisomy. The Biochemical Journal. 2010;**431**(2):299-310

[6] Valenti D, Manente GA, Moro L, Marra E, Vacca RA. Deficit of complex I activity in human skin fibroblasts with chromosome 21 trisomy and overproduction of reactive oxygen species by mitochondria: Involvement of the cAMP/PKA signalling pathway. The Biochemical Journal. 2011;**435**(3):679-688

[7] Kim SH, Vlkolinsky R, Cairns N, Fountoulakis M, Lubec G. The reduction of NADH ubiquinone oxidoreductase 24- and 75-kDa subunits in brains of patients with Down syndrome and Alzheimer's disease. Life Sciences. 2001;**68**(24):2741-2750

[8] Arbuzova S, Hutchin T, Cuckle H. Mitochondrial dysfunction and Down's syndrome. BioEssays: News and Reviews in Molecular, Cellular and Developmental Biology. 2002;**24**(8):681-684

[9] Busciglio J, Pelsman A, Wong C, Pigino G, Yuan M, Mori H, et al. Altered metabolism of the amyloid beta precursor protein is associated with mitochondrial dysfunction in Down's syndrome. Neuron. 2002;**33**(5):677-688

[10] Shukkur EA, Shimohata A, Akagi T, Yu W, Yamaguchi M, Murayama M, et al. Mitochondrial dysfunction and tau hyperphosphorylation in Ts1Cje, a mouse model for Down syndrome. Human Molecular Genetics. 2006;**15**(18):2752-2762

[11] Valenti D, de Bari L, de Rasmo D, Signorile A, Henrion-Caude A, Contestabile A, et al. The polyphenols resveratrol and epigallocatechin-3-gallate restore the severe impairment of mitochondria in hippocampal progenitor cells from a Down syndrome mouse model. Biochimica et Biophysica Acta. 2016;**1862**(6):1093-1104

[12] Cowley PM, Keslacy S, Middleton FA, DeRuisseau LR, Fernhall B, Kanaley JA, et al. Functional and biochemical characterization of soleus muscle in Down syndrome mice: Insight into the muscle dysfunction seen in the human condition. American Journal of Physiology Regulatory, Integrative and Comparative Physiology. 2012;**303**(12):R1251-R1260

[13] Helguera P, Seiglie J, Rodriguez J, Hanna M, Helguera G, Busciglio J. Adaptive downregulation of mitochondrial function in down syndrome. Cell Metabolism. 2013;**17**(1):132-140

[14] Tanaka A, Cleland MM, Xu S, Narendra DP, Suen DF, Karbowski M, et al. Proteasome and p97 mediate mitophagy and degradation of mitofusins induced by Parkin. The Journal of Cell Biology. 2010;**191**(7):1367-1380

[15] Westermann B. Mitochondrial fusion and fission in cell life and death. Nature Reviews Molecular Cell Biology. 2010;**11**(12):872-884

[16] Fischer F, Hamann A, Osiewacz HD. Mitochondrial quality control: An integrated network of pathways. Trends in Biochemical Sciences. 2012;**37**(7):284-292

[17] Golpich M, Amini E, Mohamed Z, Azman Ali R, Mohamed Ibrahim N, Ahmadiani A. Mitochondrial dysfunction and biogenesis in neurodegenerative diseases: Pathogenesis and treatment. CNS Neuroscience & Therapeutics. 2017;**23**(1):5-22

[18] Leone TC, Lehman JJ, Finck BN, Schaeffer PJ, Wende AR, Boudina S, et al. PGC-1alpha deficiency causes multi-system energy metabolic derangements: Muscle dysfunction, abnormal weight control and hepatic steatosis. PLoS Biology. 2005;**3**(4):e101

[19] Scarpulla RC. Metabolic control of mitochondrial biogenesis through the PGC-1 family regulatory network. Biochimica et Biophysica Acta. 2011;**1813**(7):1269-1278

[20] Petrozzi L, Ricci G, Giglioli NJ, Siciliano G, Mancuso M. Mitochondria and neurodegeneration. Bioscience Reports. 2007;**27**(1-3):87-104

[21] Vilardell M, Rasche A, Thormann A, Maschke-Dutz E, Perez-Jurado LA, Lehrach H, et al. Meta-analysis of heterogeneous Down syndrome data reveals consistent genome-wide dosage effects related to neurological processes. BMC Genomics. 2011;**12**:229

[22] Sturgeon X, Le T, Ahmed MM, Gardiner KJ. Pathways to cognitive deficits in Down syndrome. Progress in Brain Research. 2012;**197**:73-100

[23] Izzo A, Manco R, Bonfiglio F, Cali G, De Cristofaro T, Patergnani S, et al. NRIP1/RIP140 siRNA-mediated attenuation counteracts mitochondrial dysfunction in Down syndrome. Human Molecular Genetics. 2014;**23**(16):4406-4419

[24] Fritah A, Christian M, Parker MG. The metabolic coregulator RIP140: An update. American Journal of Physiology. Endocrinology and Metabolism. 2010;**299**(3):E335-E340

[25] Chen Y, Wang Y, Chen J, Chen X, Cao W, Chen S, et al. Roles of transcriptional corepressor RIP140 and coactivator PGC-1alpha in energy state of chronically infarcted rat hearts and mitochondrial function of cardiomyocytes. Molecular and Cellular Endocrinology. 2012;**362**(1-2):11-18

[26] Robinson-Rechavi M, Escriva Garcia H, Laudet V. The nuclear receptor superfamily. Journal of Cell Science. 2003;**116**(Pt 4):585-586

[27] Lin J, Handschin C, Spiegelman BM. Metabolic control through the PGC-1 family of transcription coactivators. Cell Metabolism. 2005;**1**(6):361-370

[28] Schreiber SN, Emter R, Hock MB, Knutti D, Cardenas J, Podvinec M, et al. The estrogen-related receptor alpha (ERRalpha) functions in PPARgamma coactivator 1alpha (PGC-1alpha)-induced mitochondrial biogenesis. Proceedings of the National Academy of Sciences of the United States of America. 2004;**101**(17):6472-6477

[29] De Cegli R, Romito A, Iacobacci S, Mao L, Lauria M, Fedele AO, et al. A mouse embryonic stem cell bank for inducible overexpression of human chromosome 21 genes. Genome Biology. 2010;**11**(6):R64

[30] Askanas V, McFerrin J, Baque S, Alvarez RB, Sarkozi E, Engel WK. Transfer of beta-amyloid precursor protein gene using adenovirus vector causes mitochondrial abnormalities in cultured normal human muscle. Proceedings of the National Academy of Sciences of the United States of America. 1996;**93**(3):1314-1319

[31] Bartley MG, Marquardt K, Kirchhof D, Wilkins HM, Patterson D, Linseman DA. Overexpression of amyloid-beta protein precursor induces mitochondrial oxidative stress and activates the intrinsic apoptotic cascade. Journal of Alzheimer's Disease: JAD. 2012;**28**(4):855-868

[32] Chen JX, Yan SS. Role of mitochondrial amyloid-beta in Alzheimer's disease. Journal of Alzheimer's Disease: JAD. 2010;**20**(Suppl 2):S569-S578

[33] Demuro A, Parker I, Stutzmann GE. Calcium signaling and amyloid toxicity in Alzheimer disease. The Journal of Biological Chemistry. 2010;**285**(17):12463-12468

[34] Manczak M, Mao P, Calkins MJ, Cornea A, Reddy AP, Murphy MP, et al. Mitochondria-targeted antioxidants protect against amyloid-beta toxicity in Alzheimer's disease neurons. Journal of Alzheimer's Disease: JAD. 2010;**20**(Suppl 2):S609-S631

[35] Anandatheerthavarada HK, Biswas G, Robin MA, Avadhani NG. Mitochondrial targeting and a novel transmembrane arrest of Alzheimer's amyloid precursor protein impairs mitochondrial function in neuronal cells. The Journal of Cell Biology. 2003;**161**(1):41-54

[36] Lu J, Esposito G, Scuderi C, Steardo L, Delli-Bovi LC, Hecht JL, et al. S100B and APP promote a gliocentric shift and impaired neurogenesis in Down syndrome neural progenitors. PLoS One. 2011;**6**(7):e22126

[37] Rytinki MM, Palvimo JJ. SUMOylation modulates the transcription repressor function of RIP140. The Journal of Biological Chemistry. 2008;**283**(17):11586-11595

[38] Rytinki MM, Palvimo JJ. SUMOylation attenuates the function of PGC-1alpha. The Journal of Biological Chemistry. 2009;**284**(38):26184-26193

[39] de la Luna S, Estivill X. Cooperation to amplify gene-dosage-imbalance effects. Trends in Molecular Medicine. 2006;**12**(10):451-454

[40] Arron JR, Winslow MM, Polleri A, Chang CP, Wu H, Gao X, et al. NFAT dysregulation by increased dosage of DSCR1 and DYRK1A on chromosome 21. Nature. 2006;**441**(7093): 595-600

[41] Handschin C, Rhee J, Lin J, Tarr PT, Spiegelman BM. An autoregulatory loop controls peroxisome proliferator-activated receptor gamma coactivator 1alpha expression in muscle. Proceedings of the National Academy of Sciences of the United States of America. 2003;**100**(12):7111-7116

[42] Wu Y, Song W. Regulation of RCAN1 translation and its role in oxidative stress-induced apoptosis. FASEB Journal: Official Publication of the Federation of American Societies for Experimental Biology. 2013;**27**(1):208-221

[43] Chang KT, Min KT. *Drosophila melanogaster* homolog of Down syndrome critical region 1 is critical for mitochondrial function. Nature Neuroscience. 2005;**8**(11):1577-1585

[44] Peiris H, Dubach D, Jessup CF, Unterweger P, Raghupathi R, Muyderman H, et al. RCAN1 regulates mitochondrial function and increases susceptibility to oxidative stress in mammalian cells. Oxidative Medicine and Cellular Longevity. 2014;**2014**:520316

[45] Ermak G, Sojitra S, Yin F, Cadenas E, Cuervo AM, Davies KJ. Chronic expression of RCAN1-1L protein induces mitochondrial autophagy and metabolic shift from oxidative phosphorylation to glycolysis in neuronal cells. The Journal of Biological Chemistry. 2012;**287**(17):14088-14098

[46] Sun X, Wu Y, Herculano B, Song W. RCAN1 overexpression exacerbates calcium overloading-induced neuronal apoptosis. PLoS One. 2014;**9**(4):e95471

[47] Yamato F, Takaya J, Yasuhara A, Teraguchi M, Ikemoto Y, Kaneko K. Elevated intracellular calcium in neutrophils in patients with Down syndrome. Pediatrics International: Official Journal of the Japan Pediatric Society. 2009;**51**(4):474-477

[48] Wong H, Levenga J, Cain P, Rothermel B, Klann E, Hoeffer C. RCAN1 overexpression promotes age-dependent mitochondrial dysregulation related to neurodegeneration in Alzheimer's disease. Acta Neuropathologica. 2015;**130**(6):829-843

[49] Duan H, Li Y, Yan L, Yang H, Wu J, Qian P, et al. Rcan1-1L overexpression induces mitochondrial autophagy and improves cell survival in angiotensin II-exposed cardiomyocytes. Experimental Cell Research. 2015;**335**(1):99-106

[50] Groner Y, Elroy-Stein O, Avraham KB, Schickler M, Knobler H, Minc-Golomb D, et al. Cell damage by excess CuZnSOD and Down's syndrome. Biomedicine & Pharmacotherapy = Biomedecine & Pharmacotherapie. 1994;**48**(5-6):231-240

[51] Fridovich I. Superoxide radical and superoxide dismutases. Annual Review of Biochemistry. 1995;**64**:97-112

[52] Wolvetang EJ, Wilson TJ, Sanij E, Busciglio J, Hatzistavrou T, Seth A, et al. ETS2 overexpression in transgenic models and in Down syndrome predisposes to apoptosis via the p53 pathway. Human Molecular Genetics. 2003;**12**(3):247-255

[53] Helguera P, Pelsman A, Pigino G, Wolvetang E, Head E, Busciglio J. ets-2 promotes the activation of a mitochondrial death pathway in Down's syndrome neurons. The Journal of Neuroscience: The Official Journal of the Society for Neuroscience. 2005;**25**(9):2295-2303

[54] Predescu SA, Predescu DN, Knezevic I, Klein IK, Malik AB. Intersectin-1s regulates the mitochondrial apoptotic pathway in endothelial cells. The Journal of Biological Chemistry. 2007;**282**(23):17166-17178

[55] Ferretti E, Villaescusa JC, Di Rosa P, Fernandez-Diaz LC, Longobardi E, Mazzieri R, et al. Hypomorphic mutation of the TALE gene Prep1 (pKnox1) causes a major reduction of Pbx and Meis proteins and a pleiotropic embryonic phenotype. Molecular and Cellular Biology. 2006;**26**(15):5650-5662

[56] Kanzleiter T, Rath M, Penkov D, Puchkov D, Schulz N, Blasi F, et al. Pknox1/Prep1 regulates mitochondrial oxidative phosphorylation components in skeletal muscle. Molecular and Cellular Biology. 2014;**34**(2):290-298

[57] Fan M, Rhee J, St-Pierre J, Handschin C, Puigserver P, Lin J, et al. Suppression of mitochondrial respiration through recruitment of p160 myb binding protein to PGC-1alpha: Modulation by p38 MAPK. Genes & Development. 2004;**18**(3):278-289

[58] Di Domenico F, Pupo G, Mancuso C, Barone E, Paolini F, Arena A, et al. Bach1 overexpression in Down syndrome correlates with the alteration of the HO-1/BVR-a system: Insights for transition to Alzheimer's disease. Journal of Alzheimer's Disease: JAD. 2015;**44**(4):1107-1120

[59] Marshak DR, Pena LA. Potential role of S100 beta in Alzheimer's disease: An hypothesis involving mitotic protein kinases. Progress in Clinical and Biological Research. 1992;**379**:289-307

[60] Muller CM, Akhavan AC, Bette M. Possible role of S-100 in glia-neuronal signalling involved in activity-dependent plasticity in the developing mammalian cortex. Journal of Chemical Neuroanatomy. 1993;**6**(4):215-227

[61] Yan W, Wilson CC, Haring JH. 5-HT1a receptors mediate the neurotrophic effect of serotonin on developing dentate granule cells. Brain Research Developmental Brain Research. 1997;**98**(2):185-190

[62] Mariggio MA, Fulle S, Calissano P, Nicoletti I, Fano G. The brain protein S-100ab induces apoptosis in PC12 cells. Neuroscience. 1994;**60**(1):29-35

[63] Allore R, O'Hanlon D, Price R, Neilson K, Willard HF, Cox DR, et al. Gene encoding the beta subunit of S100 protein is on chromosome 21: Implications for Down syndrome. Science. 1988;**239**(4845):1311-1313

[64] Shapiro LA, Bialowas-McGoey LA, Whitaker-Azmitia PM. Effects of S100B on serotonergic plasticity and neuroinflammation in the hippocampus in down syndrome and Alzheimer's disease: Studies in an S100B overexpressing mouse model. Cardiovascular Psychiatry and Neurology. 2010;**2010**

[65] Esposito G, Imitola J, Lu J, De Filippis D, Scuderi C, Ganesh VS, et al. Genomic and functional profiling of human Down syndrome neural progenitors implicates S100B and aquaporin 4 in cell injury. Human Molecular Genetics. 2008;**17**(3):440-457

[66] Letourneau A, Antonarakis SE. Genomic determinants in the phenotypic variability of Down syndrome. Progress in Brain Research. 2012;**197**:15-28

[67] Quinones-Lombrana A, Blanco JG. Chromosome 21-derived hsa-miR-155-5p regulates mitochondrial biogenesis by targeting Mitochondrial Transcription Factor A (TFAM). Biochimica et Biophysica Acta. 2015;**1852**(7):1420-1427

[68] Izzo A, Manco R, de Cristofaro T, Bonfiglio F, Cicatiello R, Mollo N, et al. Over-expression of chromosome 21 miRNAs may affect mitochondrial function in the hearts of Down syndrome fetuses. International Journal of Genomics. 2017 In press

[69] Tokumaru S, Suzuki M, Yamada H, Nagino M, Takahashi T. Let-7 regulates Dicer expression and constitutes a negative feedback loop. Carcinogenesis. 2008;**29**(11):2073-2077

[70] Cisterna B, Costanzo M, Scherini E, Zancanaro C, Malatesta M. Ultrastructural features of skeletal muscle in adult and aging Ts65Dn mice, a murine model of Down syndrome. Muscles, Ligaments and Tendons Journal. 2013;**3**(4):287-294

[71] Romanello V, Guadagnin E, Gomes L, Roder I, Sandri C, Petersen Y, et al. Mitochondrial fission and remodelling contributes to muscle atrophy. The EMBO Journal. 2010;**29**(10): 1774-1785

[72] Romanello V, Sandri M. Mitochondrial biogenesis and fragmentation as regulators of muscle protein degradation. Current Hypertension Reports. 2010;**12**(6):433-439

[73] Soriano FX, Liesa M, Bach D, Chan DC, Palacin M, Zorzano A. Evidence for a mitochondrial regulatory pathway defined by peroxisome proliferator-activated receptor-gamma coactivator-1 alpha, estrogen-related receptor-alpha, and mitofusin 2. Diabetes. 2006;**55**(6):1783-1791

[74] Roth GM, Sun B, Greensite FS, Lott IT, Dietrich RB. Premature aging in persons with Down syndrome: MR findings. AJNR American Journal of Neuroradiology. 1996;**17**(7):1283-1289

[75] Nakamura E, Tanaka S. Biological ages of adult men and women with Down's syndrome and its changes with aging. Mechanisms of Ageing and Development. 1998;**105**(1-2): 89-103

[76] Angelopoulou N, Matziari C, Tsimaras V, Sakadamis A, Souftas V, Mandroukas K. Bone mineral density and muscle strength in young men with mental retardation (with and without Down syndrome). Calcified Tissue International. 2000;**66**(3):176-180

[77] Thompson LV. Age-related muscle dysfunction. Experimental Gerontology. 2009;**44**(1-2): 106-111

[78] Busciglio J, Yankner BA. Apoptosis and increased generation of reactive oxygen species in Down's syndrome neurons in vitro. Nature. 1995;**378**(6559):776-779

[79] Cenini G, Dowling AL, Beckett TL, Barone E, Mancuso C, Murphy MP, et al. Association between frontal cortex oxidative damage and beta-amyloid as a function of age in Down syndrome. Biochimica et Biophysica Acta. 2012;**1822**(2):130-138

[80] Oettinghaus B, Schulz JM, Restelli LM, Licci M, Savoia C, Schmidt A, et al. Synaptic dysfunction, memory deficits and hippocampal atrophy due to ablation of mitochondrial fission in adult forebrain neurons. Cell Death and Differentiation. 2016;**23**(1):18-28

[81] Emerit J, Edeas M, Bricaire F. Neurodegenerative diseases and oxidative stress. Biomedicine & Pharmacotherapy = Biomedecine & Pharmacotherapie. 2004;**58**(1):39-46

[82] Hroudova J, Singh N, Fisar Z. Mitochondrial dysfunctions in neurodegenerative diseases: Relevance to Alzheimer's disease. BioMed Research International. 2014;**2014**:175062

[83] Zigman WB, Devenny DA, SJ K-MH, Jenkins EC, Urv TK, Wegiel J, et al. Alzheimer's disease in adults with down syndrome. International Review of Research in Mental Retardation. 2008;**36**:103-145

[84] Head E, Silverman W, Patterson D, Lott IT. Aging and down syndrome. Current Gerontology and Geriatrics Research. 2012;**2012**:412536

[85] Dumont M, Beal MF. Neuroprotective strategies involving ROS in Alzheimer disease. Free Radical Biology & Medicine. 2011;**51**(5):1014-1026

[86] Misonou H, Morishima-Kawashima M, Ihara Y. Oxidative stress induces intracellular accumulation of amyloid beta-protein (Abeta) in human neuroblastoma cells. Biochemistry. 2000;**39**(23):6951-6959

[87] Bertholet AM, Delerue T, Millet AM, Moulis MF, David C, Daloyau M, et al. Mitochondrial fusion/fission dynamics in neurodegeneration and neuronal plasticity. Neurobiology of Disease. 2016;**90**:3-19

[88] Ferencz C, Neill CA, Boughman JA, Rubin JD, Brenner JI, Perry LW. Congenital cardiovascular malformations associated with chromosome abnormalities: An epidemiologic study. The Journal of Pediatrics. 1989;**114**(1):79-86

[89] Park SC, Mathews RA, Zuberbuhler JR, Rowe RD, Neches WH, Lenox CC. Down syndrome with congenital heart malformation. American Journal of Diseases of Children. 1977;**131**(1):29-33

[90] Bushdid PB, Osinska H, Waclaw RR, Molkentin JD, Yutzey KE. NFATc3 and NFATc4 are required for cardiac development and mitochondrial function. Circulation Research. 2003;**92**(12):1305-1313

[91] de la Pompa JL, Timmerman LA, Takimoto H, Yoshida H, Elia AJ, Samper E, et al. Role of the NF-ATc transcription factor in morphogenesis of cardiac valves and septum. Nature. 1998;**392**(6672):182-186

[92] Graef IA, Chen F, Crabtree GR. NFAT signaling in vertebrate development. Current Opinion in Genetics & Development. 2001;**11**(5):505-512

[93] Wust RC, de Vries HJ, Wintjes LT, Rodenburg RJ, Niessen HW, Stienen GJ. Mitochondrial complex I dysfunction and altered NAD(P)H kinetics in rat myocardium in cardiac right ventricular hypertrophy and failure. Cardiovascular Research. 2016;**111**(4):362-372

[94] Fritah A, Steel JH, Nichol D, Parker N, Williams S, Price A, et al. Elevated expression of the metabolic regulator receptor-interacting protein 140 results in cardiac hypertrophy and impaired cardiac function. Cardiovascular Research. 2010;**86**(3):443-451

[95] Seok HY, Chen J, Kataoka M, Huang ZP, Ding J, Yan J, et al. Loss of MicroRNA-155 protects the heart from pathological cardiac hypertrophy. Circulation Research. 2014; **114**(10):1585-1595

[96] Grammatikopoulou MG, Manai A, Tsigga M, Tsiligiroglou-Fachantidou A, Galli-Tsinopoulou A, Zakas A. Nutrient intake and anthropometry in children and adolescents with Down syndrome—A preliminary study. Developmental Neurorehabilitation. 2008;**11**(4):260-267

[97] Lowell BB, Shulman GI. Mitochondrial dysfunction and type 2 diabetes. Science. 2005;**307**(5708):384-387

[98] Ritov VB, Menshikova EV, He J, Ferrell RE, Goodpaster BH, Kelley DE. Deficiency of subsarcolemmal mitochondria in obesity and type 2 diabetes. Diabetes. 2005;**54**(1):8-14

[99] Kelley DE, He J, Menshikova EV, Ritov VB. Dysfunction of mitochondria in human skeletal muscle in type 2 diabetes. Diabetes. 2002;**51**(10):2944-2950

[100] Hallberg M, Morganstein DL, Kiskinis E, Shah K, Kralli A, Dilworth SM, et al. A functional interaction between RIP140 and PGC-1alpha regulates the expression of the lipid droplet protein CIDEA. Molecular Cell Biology. 2008;**28**(22):6785-6795

[101] Fritah A, Steel JH, Parker N, Nikolopoulou E, Christian M, Carling D, et al. Absence of RIP140 reveals a pathway regulating glut4-dependent glucose uptake in oxidative skeletal muscle through UCP1-mediated activation of AMPK. PLoS One. 2012;**7**(2):e32520

[102] Leonardsson G, Steel JH, Christian M, Pocock V, Milligan S, Bell J, et al. Nuclear receptor corepressor RIP140 regulates fat accumulation. Proceedings of the National Academy of Sciences of the United States of America. 2004;**101**(22):8437-8442

[103] Bach D, Pich S, Soriano FX, Vega N, Baumgartner B, Oriola J, et al. Mitofusin-2 determines mitochondrial network architecture and mitochondrial metabolism. A novel regulatory mechanism altered in obesity. The Journal of Biological Chemistry. 2003;**278**(19):17190-17197

[104] Walder K, Kerr-Bayles L, Civitarese A, Jowett J, Curran J, Elliott K, et al. The mitochondrial rhomboid protease PSARL is a new candidate gene for type 2 diabetes. Diabetologia. 2005;**48**(3):459-468

[105] Turner S, Sloper P, Cunningham C, Knussen C. Health problems in children with Down's syndrome. Child: Care, Health and Development. 1990;**16**(2):83-97

[106] Selikowitz M. Health problems and health checks in school-aged children with Down syndrome. Journal of Paediatrics and Child Health. 1992;**28**(5):383-386

[107] Cruz NV, Mahmoud SA, Chen H, Lowery-Nordberg M, Berlin K, Bahna SL. Follow-up study of immune defects in patients with dysmorphic disorders. Annals of Allergy, Asthma & Immunology: Official Publication of the American College of Allergy, Asthma & Immunology. 2009;**102**(5):426-431

[108] van Trotsenburg AS, Kempers MJ, Endert E, Tijssen JG, de Vijlder JJ, Vulsma T. Trisomy 21 causes persistent congenital hypothyroidism presumably of thyroidal origin. Thyroid: Official Journal of the American Thyroid Association. 2006;**16**(7):671-680

[109] Zachor DA, Mroczek-Musulman E, Brown P. Prevalence of celiac disease in Down syndrome in the United States. Journal of Pediatric Gastroenterology and Nutrition. 2000;**31**(3):275-279

[110] Sanchez-Albisua I, Storm W, Wascher I, Stern M. How frequent is coeliac disease in Down syndrome? European Journal of Pediatrics. 2002;**161**(12):683-684

[111] Kusters MA, Verstegen RH, Gemen EF, de Vries E. Intrinsic defect of the immune system in children with Down syndrome: A review. Clinical and Experimental Immunology. 2009;**156**(2):189-193

[112] de Hingh YC, van der Vossen PW, Gemen EF, Mulder AB, Hop WC, Brus F, et al. Intrinsic abnormalities of lymphocyte counts in children with down syndrome. The Journal of Pediatrics. 2005;**147**(6):744-747

[113] Aburawi EH, Souid AK. Lymphocyte respiration in children with Trisomy 21. BMC Pediatrics. 2012;**12**:193

[114] Campello S, Lacalle RA, Bettella M, Manes S, Scorrano L, Viola A. Orchestration of lymphocyte chemotaxis by mitochondrial dynamics. The Journal of Experimental Medicine. 2006;**203**(13):2879-2886

[115] Buck MD, O'Sullivan D, Klein Geltink RI, Curtis JD, Chang CH, Sanin DE, et al. Mitochondrial dynamics controls T cell fate through metabolic programming. Cell. 2016;**166**(1):63-76

[116] de la Torre R, Dierssen M. Therapeutic approaches in the improvement of cognitive performance in Down syndrome: past, present, and future. Progress in Brain Research. 2012;**197**:1-14

[117] Costa AC, Scott-McKean JJ. Prospects for improving brain function in individuals with Down syndrome. CNS Drugs. 2013;**27**(9):679-702

[118] Gardiner KJ. Pharmacological approaches to improving cognitive function in Down syndrome: Current status and considerations. Drug Design, Development and Therapy. 2015;**9**:103-125

[119] Rodgers JT, Lerin C, Haas W, Gygi SP, Spiegelman BM, Puigserver P. Nutrient control of glucose homeostasis through a complex of PGC-1alpha and SIRT1. Nature. 2005;**434**(7029):113-118

[120] Dong W, Gao D, Zhang X. Mitochondria biogenesis induced by resveratrol against brain ischemic stroke. Medical Hypotheses. 2007;**69**(3):700-701

[121] Lagouge M, Argmann C, Gerhart-Hines Z, Meziane H, Lerin C, Daussin F, et al. Resveratrol improves mitochondrial function and protects against metabolic disease by activating SIRT1 and PGC-1alpha. Cell. 2006;**127**(6):1109-1122

[122] Jager S, Handschin C, St-Pierre J, Spiegelman BM. AMP-activated protein kinase (AMPK) action in skeletal muscle via direct phosphorylation of PGC-1alpha. Proceedings of the National Academy of Sciences of the United States of America. 2007;**104**(29):12017-12022

[123] Nicolakakis N, Aboulkassim T, Ongali B, Lecrux C, Fernandes P, Rosa-Neto P, et al. Complete rescue of cerebrovascular function in aged Alzheimer's disease transgenic mice by antioxidants and pioglitazone, a peroxisome proliferator-activated receptor gamma agonist. The Journal of Neuroscience: The Official Journal of the Society for Neuroscience. 2008;**28**(37):9287-9296

[124] Escribano L, Simon AM, Perez-Mediavilla A, Salazar-Colocho P, Del Rio J, Frechilla D. Rosiglitazone reverses memory decline and hippocampal glucocorticoid receptor down-regulation in an Alzheimer's disease mouse model. Biochemical and Biophysical Research Communications. 2009;**379**(2):406-410

[125] Johri A, Calingasan NY, Hennessey TM, Sharma A, Yang L, Wille E, et al. Pharmacologic activation of mitochondrial biogenesis exerts widespread beneficial effects in a transgenic mouse model of Huntington's disease. Human Molecular Genetics. 2012; **21**(5):1124-1137

[126] Yamaguchi S, Li H, Purevsuren J, Yamada K, Furui M, Takahashi T, et al. Bezafibrate can be a new treatment option for mitochondrial fatty acid oxidation disorders: Evaluation by in vitro probe acylcarnitine assay. Molecular Genetics and Metabolism. 2012;**107**(1-2):87-91

[127] Canto C, Auwerx J. PGC-1alpha, SIRT1 and AMPK, an energy sensing network that controls energy expenditure. Current Opinion in Lipidology. 2009;**20**(2):98-105

[128] Hofer A, Noe N, Tischner C, Kladt N, Lellek V, Schauss A, et al. Defining the action spectrum of potential PGC-1alpha activators on a mitochondrial and cellular level in vivo. Human Molecular Genetics. 2014;**23**(9):2400-2415

[129] Lott IT, Doran E, Nguyen VQ, Tournay A, Head E, Gillen DL. Down syndrome and dementia: A randomized, controlled trial of antioxidant supplementation. American Journal of Medical Genetics. Part A. 2011;**155A**(8):1939-1948

[130] Miles MV, Patterson BJ, Chalfonte-Evans ML, Horn PS, Hickey FJ, Schapiro MB, et al. Coenzyme Q10 (ubiquinol-10) supplementation improves oxidative imbalance in children with trisomy 21. Pediatric Neurology. 2007;**37**(6):398-403

[131] Ellis JM, Tan HK, Gilbert RE, Muller DP, Henley W, Moy R, et al. Supplementation with antioxidants and folinic acid for children with Down's syndrome: Randomised controlled trial. BMJ. 2008;**336**(7644):594-597

[132] Reynolds T. Antioxidants do not improve early childhood development in children with Down's syndrome. The Journal of Pediatrics. 2008;**153**(3):441

[133] Sano M, Aisen PS, Andrews HF, Tsai WY, Lai F, Dalton AJ, et al. Vitamin E in aging persons with Down syndrome: A randomized, placebo-controlled clinical trial. Neurology. 2016;**86**(22):2071-2076

[134] Littarru GP, Tiano L. Clinical aspects of coenzyme Q10: An update. Nutrition. 2010; **26**(3):250-254

[135] Uberos J, Romero J, Molina-Carballo A, Munoz-Hoyos A. Melatonin and elimination of kynurenines in children with Down's syndrome. Journal of Pediatric Endocrinology & Metabolism: JPEM. 2010;**23**(3):277-282

[136] Parisotto EB, Vidal V, Garcia-Cerro S, Lantigua S, Wilhelm Filho D, Sanchez-Barcelo EJ, et al. Chronic melatonin administration reduced oxidative damage and cellular senescence in the hippocampus of a mouse model of down syndrome. Neurochemical Research. 2016;**41**(11):2904-2913

[137] Corrales A, Parisotto EB, Vidal V, Garcia-Cerro S, Lantigua S, Diego M, et al. Pre- and post-natal melatonin administration partially regulates brain oxidative stress but does not improve cognitive or histological alterations in the Ts65Dn mouse model of Down syndrome. Behavioural Brain Research. 2017;**334**:142-154

[138] Schroeder EK, Kelsey NA, Doyle J, Breed E, Bouchard RJ, Loucks FA, et al. Green tea epigallocatechin 3-gallate accumulates in mitochondria and displays a selective antiapoptotic effect against inducers of mitochondrial oxidative stress in neurons. Antioxidants & Redox Signaling. 2009;**11**(3):469-480

[139] Srividhya R, Zarkovic K, Stroser M, Waeg G, Zarkovic N, Kalaiselvi P. Mitochondrial alterations in aging rat brain: Effective role of (−)-epigallo catechin gallate. International Journal of Developmental Neuroscience: The Official Journal of the International Society for Developmental Neuroscience. 2009;**27**(3):223-231

[140] Rezai-Zadeh K, Shytle D, Sun N, Mori T, Hou H, Jeanniton D, et al. Green tea epigallocatechin-3-gallate (EGCG) modulates amyloid precursor protein cleavage and reduces cerebral amyloidosis in Alzheimer transgenic mice. The Journal of Neuroscience: The Official Journal of the Society for Neuroscience. 2005;**25**(38):8807-8814

[141] Dragicevic N, Smith A, Lin X, Yuan F, Copes N, Delic V, et al. Green tea epigallocatechin-3-gallate (EGCG) and other flavonoids reduce Alzheimer's amyloid-induced mitochondrial dysfunction. Journal of Alzheimer's Disease: JAD. 2011;**26**(3):507-521

[142] Feng Y, Wu J, Chen L, Luo C, Shen X, Chen K, et al. A fluorometric assay of SIRT1 deacetylation activity through quantification of nicotinamide adenine dinucleotide. Analytical Biochemistry. 2009;**395**(2):205-210

[143] Alvarez E, Campos-Toimil M, Justiniano-Basaran H, Lugnier C, Orallo F. Study of the mechanisms involved in the vasorelaxation induced by (−)-epigallocatechin-3-gallate in rat aorta. British Journal of Pharmacology. 2006;**147**(3):269-280

[144] Ok WJ, Cho HJ, Kim HH, Lee DH, Kang HY, Kwon HW, et al. Epigallocatechin-3-gallate has an anti-platelet effect in a cyclic AMP-dependent manner. Journal of Atherosclerosis and Thrombosis. 2012;**19**(4):337-348

[145] Guedj F, Sebrie C, Rivals I, Ledru A, Paly E, Bizot JC, et al. Green tea polyphenols rescue of brain defects induced by overexpression of DYRK1A. PLoS One. 2009;**4**(2):e4606

[146] Valenti D, De Rasmo D, Signorile A, Rossi L, de Bari L, Scala I, et al. Epigallocatechin-3-gallate prevents oxidative phosphorylation deficit and promotes mitochondrial biogenesis in human cells from subjects with Down's syndrome. Biochimica et Biophysica Acta. 2013;**1832**(4):542-552

[147] De la Torre R, De Sola S, Pons M, Duchon A, de Lagran MM, Farre M, et al. Epigallocatechin-3-gallate, a DYRK1A inhibitor, rescues cognitive deficits in Down syndrome mouse models and in humans. Molecular Nutrition & Food Research. 2014;**58**(2):278-288

[148] Stagni F, Giacomini A, Emili M, Trazzi S, Guidi S, Sassi M, et al. Short- and long-term effects of neonatal pharmacotherapy with epigallocatechin-3-gallate on hippocampal development in the Ts65Dn mouse model of Down syndrome. Neuroscience. 2016;**333**:277-301

[149] McElyea SD, Starbuck JM, Tumbleson-Brink DM, Harrington E, Blazek JD, Ghoneima A, et al. Influence of prenatal EGCG treatment and Dyrk1a dosage reduction on craniofacial features associated with Down syndrome. Human Molecular Genetics. 2016;**25**(22):4856-4869

[150] Stringer M, Abeysekera I, Thomas J, LaCombe J, Stancombe K, Stewart RJ, et al. Epigallocatechin-3-gallate (EGCG) consumption in the Ts65Dn model of Down syndrome fails to improve behavioral deficits and is detrimental to skeletal phenotypes. Physiology & Behavior. 2017;**177**:230-241

[151] Qanungo S, Das M, Haldar S, Basu A. Epigallocatechin-3-gallate induces mitochondrial membrane depolarization and caspase-dependent apoptosis in pancreatic cancer cells. Carcinogenesis. 2005;**26**(5):958-967

[152] Kim HS, Quon MJ, Kim JA. New insights into the mechanisms of polyphenols beyond antioxidant properties; lessons from the green tea polyphenol, epigallocatechin 3-gallate. Redox Biology. 2014;**2**:187-195

[153] Porquet D, Casadesus G, Bayod S, Vicente A, Canudas AM, Vilaplana J, et al. Dietary resveratrol prevents Alzheimer's markers and increases life span in SAMP8. Age. 2013;**35**(5):1851-1865

[154] Alagiakrishnan K, Sankaralingam S, Ghosh M, Mereu L, Senior P. Antidiabetic drugs and their potential role in treating mild cognitive impairment and Alzheimer's disease. Discovery Medicine. 2013;**16**(90):277-286

[155] Caton PW, Nayuni NK, Kieswich J, Khan NQ, Yaqoob MM, Corder R. Metformin suppresses hepatic gluconeogenesis through induction of SIRT1 and GCN5. The Journal of Endocrinology. 2010;**205**(1):97-106

[156] Wang J, Gallagher D, DeVito LM, Cancino GI, Tsui D, He L, et al. Metformin activates an atypical PKC-CBP pathway to promote neurogenesis and enhance spatial memory formation. Cell Stem Cell. 2012;**11**(1):23-35

[157] Salomaki H, Vahatalo LH, Laurila K, Jappinen NT, Penttinen AM, Ailanen L, et al. Prenatal metformin exposure in mice programs the metabolic phenotype of the offspring during a high fat diet at adulthood. PLoS One. 2013;**8**(2):e56594

[158] Labuzek K, Suchy D, Gabryel B, Bielecka A, Liber S, Okopien B. Quantification of metformin by the HPLC method in brain regions, cerebrospinal fluid and plasma of rats treated with lipopolysaccharide. Pharmacological Reports: PR. 2010;**62**(5):956-965